D1109997

Natural Alternatives

for Weight Loss

Also by Michael Murray:

Natural Alternatives for Weight Loss

Michael T. Murray, N.D.

William Morrow and Company, Inc.

New York

IMPORTANT: PLEASE READ

The information in this book is intended to increase your knowledge about natural remedies and by no means is intended to diagnose or treat an individual's health problems or ailments. The information given is not medical advice nor is it presented as a course of personalized treatment. There may be risks involved in connection with some of the natural remedies suggested in this book, just as there may be risks involved in connection with prescription drugs. Therefore, before starting any type of natural remedy or medical treatment, or before discontinuing any course of medical treatment you may now be undergoing, you should consult your own health-care practitioner.

Copyright © 1996 by Michael T. Murray
The recipes appearing on pages 44, 51, 72, 73, and 80 are from *The Good Herb* by Judith Benn Hurley. Copyright © 1995 by Judith Benn Hurley. By Permission of William Morrow and Company, Inc.

All rights reserved. No part of this book may be reproduced or utilized in any form or by any means, electronic or mechanical, including photocopying, recording, or by any information storage or retrieval system, without permission in writing from the Publisher. Inquiries should be addressed to Permissions Department, William Morrow and Company, Inc., 1350 Avenue of the Americas, New York, N.Y. 10019.

It is the policy of William Morrow and Company, Inc., and its imprints and affiliates, recognizing the importance of preserving what has been written, to print the books we publish on acid-free paper, and we exert our best efforts to that end.

Library of Congress Cataloging-in-Publication Data

Murray, Michael T.
    Natural alternatives for weight loss / Michael T. Murray.
        p.   cm.
    Includes index.
    ISBN 0-688-14685-6
    1. Weight loss.   I. Title.
RM222.2.M85   1996
613.2'5—dc20   95-43961
                                                                  CIP

PRINTED IN THE UNITED STATES OF AMERICA

FIRST EDITION

1   2   3   4   5   6   7   8   9   10

BOOK DESIGN BY LAURA HAMMOND HOUGH

Preface

A great deal of scientific research has been conducted over the past few decades in the attempt to answer two very important questions: Why do people get fat, and why can't people who are fat lose weight? The answers to these questions have led to a better understanding of the cause and effective treatment of obesity. However, despite this increased understanding, the number of Americans who are overweight continues to rise.

According to the results of a recently completed survey (the National Health and Nutrition Examination Survey III, phase 1), the number of overweight Americans has increased dramatically in the last decade. In 1980 the prevalence of obesity (defined as greater than 20 percent above the ideal weight for height) in the United States was 25.4 percent. By 1991 the rate was 33.3 percent and rising.[1]

Even more alarming has been the dramatic increase in the number of obese children in the United States noted in the last thirty years.[2,3] There are nearly twice as many fat children now compared with the early 1960s. Given the fact that childhood obesity is conclusively linked to adult obesity, the dramatic increase in childhood obesity will undoubtedly result in an even greater frequency of adult obesity as these children grow up.

Current estimates indicate that over 60 million Americans are at least 20 percent above their ideal body weight.[1] In 1990 the U.S. Department of Health unveiled the Healthy People 2000 Goals. One of the key goals was to reduce the percentage of overweight Americans to 20 percent by the turn of the century. Obviously we are not going to achieve that goal. In fact if the trend continues, over 40 percent of Americans will be obese by the year 2000.

So what is the answer to the question of why so many Americans are overweight? Of course there are many factors to consider, but the bottom line is that most Americans eat a diet high in fat and live a lifestyle in which they get little, if any, physical activity. If the cause is dietary and lifestyle practices, then the solution is to make major changes in these areas.

An Example of Successful Weight Loss

Do you know anyone who has achieved lasting weight loss? Have you ever asked him how he did it? More than likely he did it by changing his diet and lifestyle. If you do not know anyone personally who has been successful with weight loss, let me offer a role model—Oprah Winfrey.

Oprah's battle with her weight has been extremely public. You may remember that in 1988 Oprah lost sixty-seven pounds by following a 400-calorie-a-day liquid protein diet. She lost all this weight only to gain it back and more. Oprah fell into the old trap of trying to starve herself thin. This method simply does not work! The body has a built-in protective response when food intake is dramatically reduced. It dramatically slows down metabolism to avoid starvation. After being on such a restricted calorie intake, when Oprah started eating again, even if her calorie intake was normal for her weight, the slowed-down metabolism ensured rapid weight gain.

This was Oprah's weight-loss failure. Let me now tell you about her weight-loss success. In 1993 Oprah made a total commitment to being healthy. She found out what she needed to do in order to achieve a higher level of wellness. She learned that she needed to follow a diet that was high in nutrition but low in calories. She learned that she needed to exercise. Her rate of weight loss was less dramatic than it was

eginning of 1994 it had become quite
ticeably thinner figure was once again
e cover of tabloids. She had lost the
s this a short-term success or a perma-
that as long as Oprah focuses on what
she needs to do to stay healthy, she will keep the weight off.

Beating the Odds

Achieving successful and permanent weight loss is extremely difficult. Few people want to be overweight, yet according to several long-term studies, only about 5 percent of overweight individuals are able to attain and maintain "normal" body weight. You can beat the odds naturally without resorting to over-the-counter or prescription drugs. This book will help you learn more about what you can do to achieve your long-term goals for weight loss.

There are literally hundreds of diets and diet programs that claim to be the answer to the problem of obesity. Dieters are constantly bombarded with new reports of "wonder" diets to follow. Is the program I am recommending better than all of the other weight loss programs you have tried before? Yes. I know that if you follow the recommendations given in this book, you will achieve your weight loss goals.

A successful program for weight loss must be consistent with the four cornerstones of good health—proper diet, adequate exercise, a positive mental attitude, and the right support for the body through natural measures. All of these components are critical and interrelated. A successful program must incorporate these four measures, because although improvement in one facet may be enough to result in some positive changes, implementing all four will produce the greatest results. Such a program is offered here.

MICHAEL T. MURRAY, N.D.

Contents

Contents

Natural Alternatives

for Weight Loss

Chapter 1

Why Diets Don't Work

D o you want to lose weight? Then the last thing you should do is go on a diet that reduces your food intake. You will need to alter the type of foods that you choose to eat as well as possibly reducing the number of calories, but severely restricting food intake feeds into a phenomenon that too many Americans know firsthand—the yo-yo effect. They lose weight only to put it right back on and then some.

The cause of the yo-yo effect is tied to the very reason why some people are more prone to being overweight than others—*metabolism*. Most diets do not work because the focus is on restricting food intake, not on enhancing metabolism. Throughout this book you will be given recommendations that focus on turning up your metabolism to burn more calories.

Have you ever had a friend who could eat all the food she wanted and still stay thin, while sometimes it felt that if you simply looked at food, it tended to go right to your hips or midsection? The explanation you have probably heard is that it is a difference in metabolism. This answer is absolutely correct. How would you like to have the metabolism of a thin person? Is it possible? Yes, it is possible, and you will learn how.

In order fully to appreciate the program that will be recommended in the ensuing chapters, it is important that you understand what predisposes some people to a lifetime battle of the bulge.

In the Beginning

Developing a tendency to be overweight really begins at the moment of conception. Although there may or may not be a specific "obesity gene," the tendency to be overweight is definitely inherited. If one of your parents was overweight, you have an uphill battle. If both parents were overweight, it is an uphill battle with a fifty-pound backpack—a little harder, but not impossible.

Also important in determining the likelihood of developing obesity is the diet of your mother while you were still in the womb as well as your early infant nutrition. An excess of calories during this stage of development can lead to the formation of an increased number of fat cells for the rest of the baby's life. This type of obesity is referred to as hyperplastic—*hyper-* means "increased," *-plastic* means "cells." In *hyperplastic obesity* there is an increased number of fat cells throughout the body.

Because it is harder to develop new fat cells in adulthood, hyperplastic obesity usually begins in childhood. Fortunately hyperplastic obesity tends to be associated with fewer serious health effects compared with *hypertrophic obesity*. This form of obesity is characterized by an increase in the size of each individual fat cell and is linked to diabetes, heart disease, high blood pressure, and other serious disturbances of metabolism.[1]

Usually with hypertrophic obesity the fat distribution is generally around the waist. This fat-cell distribution is referred to as *male-patterned,* or *android, obesity* since it is typically seen in the obese male. If the waist is bigger around than the hips, a person is said to have android obesity. If the hips are larger, then a person has *female-patterned*, or *gynecoid, obesity.*

Psychological Aspects of Obesity

Many years ago it was thought that psychological factors were largely responsible for obesity. A popular theory proposed that overweight individuals were insensitive to internal signals for hunger and satiety while simultaneously being extremely sensitive to external stimuli (sight, smell, and taste) that can increase the appetite. The problem with this theory is that it assumes that excessive eating is the primary cause of obesity in all cases.[1] There is some validity to this theory; however, it is now thought that physiological factors play a greater role than psychological factors. In other words, being overweight is based more on biological than on psychological factors.

One source of external stimuli that has definitely been shown to be associated with obesity is television watching.[2] Television watching has been demonstrated to be linked to the onset of obesity, and there is a dose-related effect (i.e., the more TV that is watched, the greater the degree of obesity). One study of 4,771 adult women that examined the relationship between time spent watching television per week and obesity demonstrated that twice as many women who reported three or more hours of TV viewing per day were obese compared with the reference group of women who watched less than one hour of television per day.[3]

Although television watching fits very nicely with the psychological theory (increased sensitivity to external cues), there are also several physiological effects of watching TV that promote obesity, such as reducing physical activity and the actual lowering of resting (basal) metabolic rate to a level similar to that experienced during trancelike states. These factors clearly support the physiological view. In addition, exercise levels tend to be lower in people who watch a lot of TV.

Psychological Therapy

A number of psychological therapies have been tried to promote weight loss. Unfortunately there has not been a great deal of success when psychological therapies are used alone.[4] The reason why psychological therapies may fail is that their primary goal is to reduce food intake. As previously stated, this dietary practice ultimately fails. In addition, overweight individuals often consume far less calories than their lean counterparts and still put on weight. This paradox highlights the greater importance of the physiological processes that promote obesity.

Rather than using psychological therapies is the attempt to reduce food intake, my recommendation is to utilize techniques that promote a positive self-image and high self-esteem. There is a tremendous stigma attached to being overweight. As a result the overweight individual has experienced much psychological trauma. Fashion trends, insurance programs, college placements, job opportunities—all discriminate against the obese person. Consequently the obese person learns many self-defeating and self-degrading attitudes. He is led to believe that fat is "bad," which often results in a vicious cycle of low self-esteem, depression, overeating for consolation, increased fatness, social rejection, and further lowering of self-esteem.

If techniques designed to boost self-esteem and acceptance are not incorporated into a weight loss program, even the most perfect diet and exercise plan will fail. Improving the way overweight people feel about themselves may assist them in changing their eating behaviors. Techniques to raise self-esteem and boost confidence are given in the next chapter, "Making the Commitment."

A Physiological View of Obesity

Whereas the psychological theory proposed that obese individuals have a decreased sensitivity to internal cues of hunger and satisfaction, an emerging theory of obesity states almost the opposite: Obese individuals appear to be extremely sensitive to specific internal cues.[5]

The physiological theories of obesity are tied to the metabolism of the fat cells. These models support the notion that obesity is not just a matter of overeating, and explain why some people can eat very large quantities of calories and not increase their weight substantially, while for others just the reverse is true.

Research with animals and humans has found that each person has a programmed "set-point" weight.[6] The *set point* is the weight that a body tries to maintain by regulating caloric intake. It has been postulated that individual fat cells control this set point: When the fat cell becomes smaller, it sends a powerful message to the brain to eat. Since the obese individual often has both more and larger fat cells, the result is an overpowering urge to eat.

The existence of this set point explains why most diets don't work. While the obese individual can fight off the impulse to eat for a time, eventually the signal becomes too strong to ignore. The result is rebound overeating, with individuals often exceeding their previous weight. In addition, their set point is now set at a higher level, making it even more difficult to lose weight. This effect has been termed the *ratchet effect* and *yo-yo dieting*.

The set point seems to be tied to fat-cell insulin sensitivity. Obesity leads to insulin insensitivity and vice versa. Insulin is a hormone produced by the beta cells of the pancreas that increases the rate that blood sugar (glucose) is taken up by cells throughout the body. When there is a lack of insulin, or if the cells of the body have become insensitive to insulin, it results in diabetes—a chronic disorder of carbohydrate, fat, and protein metabolism characterized by fasting elevations of blood sugar (glucose) levels and a greatly increased risk of heart disease, stroke, kidney disease, and loss of nerve function. When cells become insensitive to insulin, not only is there impaired transport of blood sugar (glucose) into the cells, but there is also impaired burning of fat stores for energy. Both obesity and diabetes are strongly linked to the Western diet, presumably due to the deleterious effect saturated fats and refined carbohydrates have on internal mechanisms that control blood sugar levels.[7]

The key to overcoming the fat cell's set point appears to

be increasing the sensitivity of the fat cells to insulin. This sensitivity apparently can be improved, and the set point lowered, by exercise, a specially designed diet, and several nutritional supplements that will be discussed in later chapters. The set-point theory suggests that a diet that does not improve insulin sensitivity will most likely fail to provide long-term results.

Increasing the body's sensitivity to insulin results in less insulin being secreted. This effect is very important for several reasons. When the body's fat cells are pumped up with high levels of fat, insulin triggers the body to manufacture more fat cells. Once a fat cell is formed, it sends signals to the brain to eat so that it can be filled with fat, thereby producing a long-term stimulus to weight gain. When an overweight individual loses fat, it is from each individual fat cell. The fat cell will shrink, but never go away. The body is able to add new fat cells, but it cannot reduce the number of existing fat cells.[8]

It should be clear that the set point of the fat cells not only predispose an individual to be overweight, it also leads to an increased susceptibility to gaining weight following weight loss due to the ratchet effect. It is this physiology that is largely responsible for the ratchet effect and yo-yo dieting; however, the loss of muscle mass (the prime burner of fat in the body) caused by dieting is also a factor. Throughout this book you will learn ways to prevent the ratchet effect and yo-yo dieting by reversing the tendency of enhanced production and storage of fat. One of the key methods for achieving these goals is improving the sensitivity of the fat cells to insulin.

Syndrome X

Insulin insensitivity (also known as insulin resistance) is linked not only to obesity and diabetes but also to syndrome X. *Syndrome X* is a term used to describe the clinical condition characterized by insulin insensitivity, high blood cholesterol and triglyceride levels, elevated blood pressure, and android obesity.[9] Other terms to describe this syndrome include *the metabolic cardiovascular risk syndrome (MCVS), Reaven's syndrome, insulin resistance syndrome,* and *atherothrombogenic syndrome.* While there is a push to abandon the term *syndrome X,* it has nonetheless persisted.[10]

I find the whole discussion of syndrome X in medical textbooks and journal articles somewhat amusing. *Syndrome X* is the label that modern medicine has chosen to describe a condition clearly caused by poor dietary and lifestyle choices. The human body was simply not designed to handle the amount of refined sugar, salt, saturated fats, and other harmful food compounds that many Americans feed it. The result is that a metabolic syndrome emerges—elevated insulin levels, obesity, elevated blood cholesterol and triglycerides, and high blood pressure. Obesity, increased insulin secretion, syndrome X, and type II diabetes can be viewed as a progression of the same illness—the body's adaptation to a poor diet and lack of physical activity.

If you need to lower blood cholesterol and blood pressure, I strongly urge you to follow the recommendations in my book *Natural Alternatives to Over-the-Counter and Prescription Drugs* (Morrow, 1994). There you will learn how to effectively lower cholesterol and blood pressure levels with diet, exercise, nutritional supplements, and herbal medicines.

Diet-Induced Thermogenesis

A certain amount of the food we consume is converted immediately to heat. This is known as *diet-induced thermogenesis* (heat production). Diet-induced thermogenesis is the method in which the body "wastes" calories.

Researchers now tell us that the level of diet-induced thermogenesis is what determines whether an individual is likely to be overweight. In lean individuals a meal may stimulate up to a 40 percent increase in heat production. By contrast overweight individuals often display only a 10 percent or less increase in heat production. The food energy is stored instead of being converted to heat.[11]

A major factor for the decreased thermogenesis in overweight people is insulin insensitivity.[12] Therefore enhancing insulin sensitivity may go a long way in reestablishing "normal" thermogenesis in overweight individuals.

Another of the other main reasons for the decreased

thermogenesis in overweight individuals is impaired sympathetic nervous system activity.[13] This portion of the nervous system controls many body functions, including metabolism. In other words the reason why many overweight individuals have a "slow metabolism" is because of a lack of stimulation by the sympathetic nervous system. Several natural plant stimulants will be described in chapter 6 that can activate the sympathetic nervous system, thereby increasing the metabolic rate and thermogenesis. This increase results in weight loss by addressing one of the underlying defects in the metabolism of overweight individuals.

Researchers have also shown that even after weight loss has been achieved, individuals predisposed to obesity will still have decreased diet-induced thermogenesis compared with a lean individual.[14] It is therefore important to continue to support insulin sensitivity and proper metabolism indefinitely if weight loss is to be maintained.

Brown Fat

In addition to insulin insensitivity and reduced sympathetic nervous system activity, there is another factor that determines diet-induced thermogenesis—the amount of *brown fat* an individual has. Most fat in the body is *white fat*, which consists of an energy reserve containing fats (triglycerides) housed in one large droplet. Tissue composed of white fat will look white or pale yellow. Brown-fat cells are special fat cells that contain multiple compartments instead of the one big compartment of white fat. The triglycerides are localized in smaller droplets surrounding numerous energy-producing compartments known as *mitochondria*. An extensive blood vessel network along with the density of the mitochondria gives the tissue its brown appearance as well as its impressive capacity to burn fat. The mitochondria is to the cell what the furnace is to an old-time locomotive. Instead of burning wood or coal for energy, the mitochondria burn fat.[15]

Brown fat does not produce energy very efficiently. In other tissues of the body, including white fat, the loss of chemical energy as heat is minimized. By contrast brown fat wastes energy by burning higher amounts of fat and giving off more heat. Brown fat plays a major role in diet-induced thermogenesis.

Some theories suggest that lean people have a higher percentage of brown fat to white fat than the overweight individual. There is evidence to support this theory. The amount of brown fat in modern humans is extremely small (estimates are 0.5 to 5 percent of total body weight), but because of its profound effect on diet-induced thermogenesis, as little as one ounce of brown fat (0.1 percent of body weight) could make the difference between maintaining body weight or putting on an extra ten pounds per year.[15]

Lean individuals also tend to respond differently to excess calories than overweight individuals. In one experiment lean individuals were fattened up. In order for these subjects to maintain the excess weight, they had to increase their caloric intake by 50 percent over their previous intake.[16] The opposite appears to be the case in overweight and formerly overweight individuals. In addition to requiring fewer calories to maintain their weight, studies have shown that in order to maintain a reduced weight, formerly obese persons must restrict their food intake to approximately 25 percent less than a lean person of similar weight and body size.[17]

The Effect of a High-Fat Diet on Thermogenesis

Individuals predisposed to obesity because of decreased diet-induced thermogenesis have been shown to be extremely sensitive to marked weight gain when consuming a high-fat diet compared with lean individuals.[18] These individuals are not only more sensitive to the weight-gain promoting effects of a high-fat diet, they tend to consume much more dietary fat compared with lean individuals and they tend to exercise less. Let's take a look at this equation:

Predisposition to obesity due to decreased diet-induced thermogenesis + increased sensitivity to weight-gain promoting effects of a high-fat diet + consumption of a high-fat diet + lack of exercise = Obesity.

That a low-fat diet is essential for weight control has been proven beyond any reasonable doubt. Just consider the example of the traditional Japanese diet, which consists primarily of rice, vegetables, soy foods, and fish. Compared with the American diet, in which 40 percent of the calories come from fat, the Japanese diet typically contains less than half this amount. The rate of obesity is much lower in Japanese consuming this traditional diet. But when Japanese individuals migrate to the United States and start eating the standard American diet, the rate of obesity, as well as the risk for heart disease, diabetes, and cancer, increases dramatically.[19] The rate of obesity for Japanese people living in the United States is an incredible seven times higher than in Japan. This fact highlights the fact that obesity is not really a factor of genetics and clearly demonstrates the important role of proper food selections for health and ideal body weight.

Final Comments

After reading this chapter you may feel that you are doomed to be overweight. You may feel that life is unfair and that you were dealt a hand from a deck that was stacked against you. I urge you to not be disheartened. My reason for explaining the obstacles to permanent weight loss is so that you will understand how to overcome them. Trust me, after reading the entire book you will be excited to have finally found a solution to permanent weight loss.

Chapter 2

Making the Commitment

How committed are you to achieving your weight loss goals? What are you willing to do to lose the weight and keep it off? Hopefully your answers to these questions reflect a high degree of motivation and enthusiasm. Without commitment there can be no success. If you can absolutely commit to achieving your goal, nothing can stand in your way. However, instead of focusing on losing weight I want you to focus on achieving a higher level of health.

Most people fail to realize how important good health is until they lose it. Don't wait for this to happen. You must realize that your health is your most valuable possession. The quality of your life is tied directly to your health. Don't take your health for granted; take the necessary steps to achieve a high level of health in your life.

Obesity and Risk of Serious Disease

Being overweight is a serious health risk. Overweight individuals not only die younger than their thin counterparts, their quality of life is also poorer because they tend to suffer from a multitude of health problems related to excessive weight. High blood pressure, heart disease, diabetes, arthritis, cancer, and many other chronic diseases are associated with obesity. If you are overweight and want to be healthy, you must lose weight.[1]

In 1993 a report published in the *Journal of the American Medical Association* showed that body weight was directly related to risk of early death.[2] Previous studies examining body weight and mortality were often flawed. For example, several studies did not take into consideration whether or not a person was a smoker. Smokers tend to be thinner and die sooner than nonsmokers. They die sooner not because they are thinner, but rather because smoking is deadly. The *JAMA* study only examined nonsmokers. As apparent in the chart below, the more overweight an individual is, the greater the risk of dying prematurely.

The number-one killer of Americans is heart disease. Being overweight is a major risk factor for heart disease on its own.[2] If a person is overweight and has high blood pressure

Risk of Dying from Being Overweight—All Causes

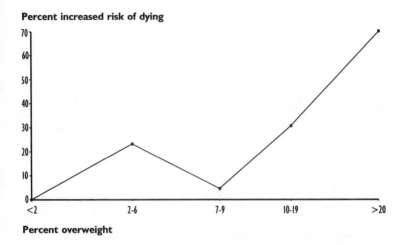

Percent increased risk of dying

Percent overweight

or high cholesterol levels, the risk is even greater. And if a person also smokes and gets little exercise, he or she is virtually a walking time bomb for a heart attack.

As stated in chapter 1, the condition that is most closely linked to being overweight is diabetes. Diabetes is divided into two major categories: type I and type II. Type I, or insulin-dependent diabetes mellitus (IDDM), occurs most often in children and adolescents. It is associated with complete destruction of the beta cells of the pancreas, which manufacture the hormone insulin. People with type I diabetes will require lifelong insulin for the control of blood sugar.

Type II, or non-insulin dependent diabetes mellitus (NIDDM), usually has an onset after forty years of age. Almost 90 percent of all diabetics are type II and approximately

Risk of Dying from Being Overweight—Diabetes

Percent increased risk of dying

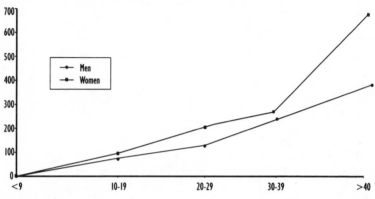

Percent overweight

90 percent of individuals with type II diabetes are obese. In type II diabetes insulin levels are typically elevated, indicating a loss of sensitivity to insulin by the cells of the body. Obesity is the major contributing factor to this loss of insulin sensitivity. Achieving ideal body weight in type II diabetics is often associated with restoration of normal blood sugar levels. In other words, achieving normal body weight will most often "cure" a person of their diabetes.

The risk of dying from diabetes is almost eight times greater in a markedly overweight person compared with someone who is at normal weight or even a few pounds above ideal body weight.[3]

If you are overweight, hopefully the information pre-

Risk of Dying from Being Overweight—Heart Disease

Percent increased risk of dying

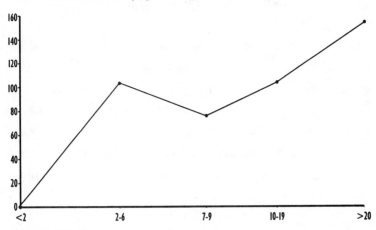

Percent overweight

sented on the stark realities of the risks you are facing for an early death will motivate you even more to lose weight. Even losing just a few pounds can have some rather remarkable effects. In one long-term study on type II diabetics it was shown that for every 2.2 pounds of weight loss life span increased by three to four months.[4] If a type II diabetic is more than twenty pounds overweight, losing that weight would mean life expectancy would be increased by a whopping 35 percent.

Taking Personal Responsibility

The first step in achieving your weight loss goals is taking personal responsibility. Take responsibility for being overweight. Do not blame it on anyone else. Do not blame it on the genes that you inherited from your parents. Do not blame it on the way that you were fed as a child. Do not blame it on your slow metabolism. Shoulder all of the responsibility. That way your focus becomes what you must do to achieve your goals.

Here is a simple, yet effective recommendation: If you want to be healthy and slim, simply make healthier choices. It sounds easy because it is easy. Many of your dietary and lifestyle choices are based on habit and marketing hype. Television, radio, newspapers, and magazines constantly bombard us with messages affecting health, diet, and lifestyle. Unfortunately much of this does not promote health. You must make a conscious effort to choose health. If you do, you will find yourself able to begin a successful weight loss program.

Enhancing Self-esteem

Increasing self-esteem and promoting a healthy positive mental attitude are critical to achieving permanent weight loss.

You will need to exercise or condition your attitude similar to the way you condition your body. Some exercises to follow are designed to help you achieve the kind of permanent results you really want by conditioning you for success. You will need to get a notebook that you can write in. This notebook will become your personal journal. A journal is a powerful tool in helping you stay in touch with your feelings, thoughts, and emotions. The exercises are designed to help you learn how to adopt healthier attitudes. These exercises will provide the foundation. Your personal journal will serve as a testimony to your success.

EXERCISE I: CREATING A POSITIVE GOAL STATEMENT

Learning to set goals in a way that results in a positive experience is critical to your success. The following guidelines can be used to set any goal, including your desired weight. You can use goal setting to create a "success cycle." Achieving goals helps you feel better about yourself, and the better you feel about yourself, the more likely you are to achieve your goals.

1. State the goal in positive terms; do not use any negative words in your goal statement. For example it is better to say "I enjoy eating healthy, low-calorie, nutritious foods" than "I will not eat sugar, candy, ice cream, and other fattening foods." Remember, always state the goal in positive terms and do not use any negative words in the goal statement.

2. Make your goal attainable and realistic. Again, goals can be used to create a success cycle and positive self-image. Little things add up to make a major difference in the way you feel about yourself.

3. Be specific. The more clearly your goal is defined, the more likely you are to reach it. What is the weight you desire? What is the body-fat percentage or measurements you desire? Clearly define what it is you want to achieve.

4. State the goal in the present tense, not the future tense. In order to reach your goal, you have to believe you have already attained it. As noted psychologist Dr. Wayne Dyer says, "You'll see it when you believe it." You must literally program yourself to achieve the goal. See and feel yourself having already achieved the goal, and success will be yours. Remember, always state your goal in the present tense.

Goal Statement

Use the guidelines above to construct a positive goal statement.

Example: "My body is strong and beautiful. I feel good about myself and my body. I am losing two pounds a week and I feel fantastic!"

Short-Term Goals

Any voyage begins with one step and is followed by many other steps. Short-term goals can be used to help you achieve those long-term results described in your positive goal statement. Get into the habit of asking yourself the following question each morning and evening: What must I do today to achieve my long-term goal?

EXERCISE 2: ASK POSITIVE QUESTIONS

According to Anthony Robbins, author of the best-sellers *Unlimited Power* and *Awakening the Giant Within,* the quality of your life is equal to the quality of the questions you habitually ask yourself. This belief is based on the assumption that whatever question you ask your brain, you will get an answer. If you want to have a better life, simply ask better questions. To help you achieve not only your desired weight but also a happier life, get into the habit of asking yourself the following questions on a consistent basis:

The Morning Questions

1. What am I most happy about in my life right now?
   Why does that make me happy?
   How does that make me feel?
2. What am I most excited about in my life right now?
   Why does that make me excited?
   How does that make me feel?
3. What am I most grateful about in my life right now?
   Why does that make me grateful?
   How does that make me feel?
4. What am I enjoying most in my life right now?
   What about that do I enjoy?
   How does that make me feel?
5. What am I committed to in my life right now?

Why am I committed to that?

How does that make me feel?

6. What must I do today to achieve my long-term goal?

The Evening Questions

1. What have I given today?

    In what ways have I been a giver today?

2. What did I learn today?

3. In what ways was today a perfect day?

4. Repeat morning questions.

The Problem of Challenge Questions

1. What is right/great about this problem?

2. What is not perfect yet?

3. What am I willing to do to make it the way I want?

4. How can I enjoy doing the things necessary to make it the way I want it?

EXERCISE 3: POSITIVE AFFIRMATIONS

An affirmation is a statement of fact that can make an imprint on the subconscious mind to create a healthy, positive self-image. In addition affirmations can actually fuel the changes you desire. Here are some guidelines for creating your own affirmations. Always phrase an affirmation in the present tense. Always phrase the affirmation in a positive way and stay tuned to the positive feelings that are generated. Keep the affirmation short and simple, but full of feeling. Be creative. Imagine yourself really experiencing what you are affirming. Make the affirmation personal and full of meaning.

Here are some examples of positive affirmations:

- I am a whole and complete person.
- I am in control of my life.
- I am an open channel of love and joy.
- I am filled with peace and wisdom.
- I am good to my body.
- I am growing stronger every day.
- I am healthier and thinner.

Using the above guidelines and examples, write down five affirmations regarding eating healthful meals and five affirmations about physical activity. State these affirmations aloud for a total of five minutes each day. Choose a location that is comfortable and quiet, and a time when you will not be interrupted or disturbed. Sit or lie in a comfortable position. Begin by taking ten deep breaths by inhaling to a count of one, holding for a count of two, and exhaling to a count of four.

EXERCISE 4: CONSTRUCT A DAILY DIARY AND CHECKLIST

In your journal you will need to enter a daily diary and a way of making sure you performed all of the daily exercises. Construct a daily checklist. Make sure you ask the morning and evening questions, write down your current weight, rewrite your goal statement, perform your affirmations. Also write down all that you consume for breakfast, lunch, snacks, dinner, as well as your physical activities, little things that made this day special, and your most successful triumph of the day.

Final Comments

Your level of commitment is the major determinant of whether or not you will be successful. Achieving your goal is accomplished by clearly identifying what it is that you want to achieve and then taking the necessary steps. To maintain a high level of commitment and motivation, a series of four exercises were described: creating a positive goal statement, asking positive questions, stating positive affirmations, and creating a daily diary and checklist.

Chapter 3

Dietary Guidelines

Perhaps the most important dietary recommendation for people trying to lose weight is to eat more. That's right, eat more. The biggest mistake people make when trying to lose weight is trying to starve themselves thin. It just doesn't work that way. As mentioned previously, most diets do not work because when the body is not fed properly, it feels that it is starving. The result: Metabolism will slow down. This slowdown means that less fat will be burned. It is clear that you must eat to lose weight. But instead of choosing high-calorie foods loaded with fats and sugars, you must eat high-fiber, low-calorie foods. These foods can help you achieve long-term results. What are high-fiber, low-calorie foods?

Vegetables, legumes (beans), most fruits, and whole grains. The importance of consuming a diet rich in these foods will be presented in this important chapter.

SEVEN USEFUL WEIGHT LOSS TIPS

1. Avoid snacking. Eat regular, planned meals. If you feel a need for a snack, drink a glass of fresh vegetable juice, eat a piece of fruit, or have a salad.
2. At all your meals eat large quantities of fresh vegetables and salads to fill you up.
3. When eating out, choose restaurants that offer low-fat choices. Avoid fast-food restaurants.
4. Drink six to eight glasses of water every day.
5. Avoid alcohol and soft drinks.
6. Learn to eat slowly. Enjoy your meals; allow your body time to realize it has been fed.
7. Avoid eating late at night, as the calories tend to be stored rather than burned for energy.

The High-Complex-Carbohydrate, High-Fiber Diet

Proper food selection is fundamental to achieving weight loss. Given the close relationship between diabetes, insulin resistance, and obesity, diets that are successful in the treatment of diabetes are the most appropriate for weight loss as well. The diet with the greatest degree of clinical support in the management of diabetes is not the one promoted by the

American Diabetes Association (ADA) but rather one popularized by Dr. James Anderson.[1] The diet is high in cereal grains, legumes, and root vegetables and restricts intake of simple sugars and fats. It is called the high-complex-carbohydrate, high-fiber diet, or HCF diet for short.

A high-complex-carbohydrate, high-fiber diet has substantial support and validation in the scientific literature as the diet of choice in the treatment of diabetes and obesity. Such a diet is also low in fat. The link between fat intake and being overweight is well accepted. People predisposed to being overweight are very efficient at storing fat calories in the body's fat-storage areas. To digest, transport, and store fat requires only 3 percent of the fat calories ingested. By contrast the metabolic pathways used by the body to convert carbohydrates to fat and then store them are "expensive" in terms of the calories that must be burned to accomplish the task. It requires 24 percent of the calories contained in carbohydrates to transform and store them as fat. Even when carbohydrates are taken to excess, the excess is generally burned up in metabolic reactions that have a tendency to increase the body's metabolic rate, not reduce it, as both high-fat and calorie-restricted diets do.[2]

Eating a diet rich in complex carbohydrates has also been shown to suppress the appetite, whereas eating a diet high in fat does not.[3] In one study of twelve overweight women, researchers found the most important variable influencing overeating was not hunger but rather the choice of foods consumed when hungry.[4] The women were provided with either a high-calorie (985 calories) or low-calorie (527 calories) lunch. At dinner the women were allowed to choose the foods they wished to consume. Analysis of dinner-meal intake revealed that when the women ate the low-calorie lunch, they overate on high fat but not high-carbohydrate foods. This study indicates that when hunger is high, it is much more tempting to eat high-fat foods. Even though there is this tendency to choose high-fat foods when hungry, your body would be better off choosing a meal low in fat and high in complex carbohydrates.

In another study by the same researchers the twelve women were once again given either a low- or high-calorie lunch. This time, however, they were assigned to receive either a high-fat or a high-carbohydrate dinner. The results were astonishing. The women consuming the high-carbohydrate dinner consumed 531 to 792 fewer calories per day than the high-fat dinner eaters regardless of whether they ate a high-calorie lunch or a low-calorie lunch.[5]

The dietary guidelines and menu suggestions given in this chapter will allow you to construct a diet low in fat but high in complex carbohydrates and fiber. Try to increase the consumption of legumes, as a high-carbohydrate, legume-rich, high-fiber diet has been shown to increase insulin sensitivity greatly in diabetics.[6]

The Healthy Exchange System

The American Dietetic Association, in conjunction with the American Diabetes Association and other groups, has developed the Exchange System, a convenient tool for the rapid estimation of the calorie, protein, fat, and carbohydrate content of a diet. Originally designed for use in creating dietary recommendations for diabetics, the exchange method is now used in the calculation of virtually all therapeutic diets. Unfortunately the ADA exchange plan does not place a strong enough focus on the quality of food choices.

The Healthy Exchange System presented here (as well as in my other books, e.g., *Encyclopedia of Natural Medicine, The Healing Power of Foods,* and *The Healing Power of Foods Cookbook*) is a healthier version because it emphasizes healthier food choices and focuses on unprocessed, whole foods. The diet is prescribed by allotting the number of exchanges allowed per list for one day. There are seven exchange lists; however, the milk and meat lists should be considered optional:

THE HEALTHY EXCHANGE SYSTEM
List 1—Vegetables
List 2—Fruits
List 3—Breads, cereals, and starchy vegetables
List 4—Legumes

List 5—Fats
List 6—Milk
List 7—Meats, fish, cheese, and eggs

Because all food portions within each exchange list provide approximately the same calories, proteins, fats, and carbohydrates per serving, it is easy to construct a diet with the proper percentages:

Carbohydrates: 65 to 75 percent of total calories
Fats: 15 to 25 percent of total calories
Protein: 10 to 15 percent of total calories
Dietary fiber: at least 50 grams

Of the carbohydrates ingested, 90 percent should be complex carbohydrates or naturally occurring sugars. Intake of refined carbohydrate and concentrated sugars (including honey, pasteurized fruit juices, and dried fruit, as well as sugar and white flour) should be limited to less than 10 percent of the total calorie intake.

Constructing a diet that meets these recommendations is simple using the exchange lists. In addition, the recommendations ensure a high intake of vital whole foods, particularly vegetables, which are rich in nutritional value.

How Many Calories Do You Need?

In determining calorie needs it is necessary to first determine ideal body weight. The most popular height and weight charts are the tables of "desirable weight" provided by the Metropolitan Life Insurance Company. The most recent edition of these tables, published in 1983, gives weight ranges for men and women at one-inch increments of height for three body-frame sizes.

1983 Metropolitan Life Insurance Height and Weight Table

Height	Weight (in pounds)		
	small frame	medium frame	large frame
Men 5'2"	128–134	131–141	138–150
5'3"	130–136	133–143	140–153
5'4"	132–138	135–145	142–156
5'5"	134–140	137–148	144–160
5'6"	136–142	139–151	146–164
5'7"	138–145	142–154	149–168
5'8"	140–148	145–157	152–172
5'9"	142–151	148–160	155–176
5'10"	144–154	151–163	158–180
5'11"	146–157	154–166	161–184
6'0"	149–160	157–170	164–188

Weights for adults ages 25 to 59 years based on lowest mortality. Weight in pounds according to frame size in indoor clothing (5 pounds for men and 3 pounds for women) wearing shoes with 1-inch heels.

1983 Metropolitan Life Insurance
Height and Weight Table (continued)

Height	Weight (in pounds)		
	small frame	medium frame	large frame
Men 6'1"	152–164	160–174	168–192
6'2"	155–168	164–178	172–197
6'3"	158–172	167–182	176–202
6'4"	162–176	171–187	181–207
Women 4'10"	102–111	109–121	118–131
4'11"	103–113	111–123	120–134
5'0"	104–115	113–126	122–137
5'1"	106–118	115–129	125–140
5'2"	108–121	118–132	128–143
5'3"	111–124	121–135	131–147
5'4"	114–127	124–138	134–151
5'5"	117–130	127–141	137–155
5'6"	120–133	130–144	140–159
5'7"	123–136	133–147	143–163
5'8"	126–139	136–150	146–167
5'9"	129–142	139–153	149–170
5'10"	132–145	142–156	152–173
5'11"	135–148	145–159	155–176
6'0"	138–151	148–162	158–179

Determining Frame Size

To make a simple determination of your frame size, extend your arm and bend the forearm upward at a ninety-degree angle. Keep the fingers straight and turn the inside of your wrist away from your body. Place the thumb and index finger of your other hand on the two prominent bones on either side of your elbow. Measure the space between your fingers with a tape measure. Compare the measurement with the following measurements for medium-framed individuals. A reading lower indicates a small frame, readings higher indicate a large frame.

	Height in 1" heels	**Elbow breadth**
Men	5'2" to 5'3"	2½" to 2⅞"
	5'4" to 5'7"	2⅝" to 2⅞"
	5'8" to 5'11"	2¾" to 3"
	6'0" to 6'3"	2¾" to 3⅛"
	6'4"	2⅞" to 3¼"
	Height in 1" heels	**Elbow breadth**
Women	4'10" to 5'3"	2¼" to 2½"
	5'4" to 5'11"	2⅜" to 2⅝"
	6'0"	2½" to 2¾"

After determining your desirable weight in pounds, convert it to kilograms by dividing it by 2.2 Next take this number and multiply it by the following calories, depending upon activity level:

Little physical activity: 30 calories
Light physical activity: 35 calories
Moderate physical activity: 40 calories
Heavy physical activity: 45 calories

Weight (in kg) × Activity Level = Approximate Calorie Requirements

$$\underline{104.5} \times \frac{30}{35} = \frac{3136}{3657}$$

The Weight Loss Equation

In order to lose one pound of fat by diet alone in one week, an individual needs to have a negative calorie intake of 500 calories per day or 3,500 calories per week since there are 3,500 calories in one pound of fat. To lose two pounds of fat each week, there must be a negative caloric balance of 1,000 calories a day. To reduce one's caloric intake by 1,000 calories per day is often difficult, as is burning an additional 1,000 calories per day by exercise (a person would need to jog for ninety minutes, play tennis for two hours, or take a brisk two-and-one-half-hour walk). The most sensible approach to weight loss is simultaneously to decrease caloric intake and to increase exercise.

Your calculation of approximate calorie requirements is probably at a level that is at least 500 calories per day less than what you are currently consuming. Since you are not likely to exercise long enough to burn off an additional 500 calories, I recommend that if you want to lose two pounds of fat per week, you reduce your calories consumed by 250 per day and burn off another 250 calories exercising. Trying to lose any more than two pounds per week is not recommended since it results in losing muscle tissue and not fat and thus will ultimately fail.

Approximate Calorie Requirement — 250 Calories =
Target Daily Calorie Intake

_____ — 250   = _____

Exchange Recommendations for Different Calorie Intakes

Now that you have your target daily calorie intake, here are recommendations from the Healthy Exchange System to construct a diet to achieve your weight loss goals. Once you have achieved your goal weight, you can increase your calorie intake to match the approximate calorie requirement for that weight.

1,500-CALORIE VEGAN DIET

List 1—Vegetables: 5 servings per day
List 2—Fruits: 2 servings per day

List 3—Breads, cereals, and starchy vegetables: 9 servings per day
List 4—Legumes: 2.5 servings per day
List 5—Fats: 4 servings per day

This recommendation would result in an intake of approximately 1,500 calories, of which 67 percent are derived from complex carbohydrates and naturally occurring sugars, 18 percent from fat, and 15 percent from protein. The protein intake is entirely from plant sources, but still provides approximately 55 grams; this number is well above the recommended daily allowance of protein intake for someone requiring 1,500 calories. At least one-half of the fat servings should be from nuts, seeds, and other whole foods from the Fat Exchange List. The dietary fiber intake would be approximately 31 to 74.5 grams.

Percentage of calories as carbohydrates: 67
Percentage of calories as fats: 18
Percentage of calories as protein: 15
Protein content: 55 g
Dietary fiber content: 31–74.5 g

1,500-CALORIE OMNIVORE DIET
List 1—Vegetables: 5 servings per day
List 2—Fruits: 2.5 servings per day
List 3—Breads, cereals, and starchy vegetables: 6 servings per day

List 4—Legumes: 1 serving per day

List 5—Fats: 5 servings per day

List 6—Milk: 1 serving per day

List 7—Meats, fish, cheese, and eggs: 2 servings per day

Percentage of calories as carbohydrates: 67

Percentage of calories as fats: 18

Percentage of calories as protein: 15

Protein content: 61 g (75% from plant sources)

Dietary fiber content: 19.5–53.5 g

2,000-CALORIE VEGAN DIET

List 1—Vegetables: 5.5 servings per day

List 2—Fruits: 2 servings per day

List 3—Breads, cereals, and starchy vegetables: 11 servings per day

List 4—Legumes: 5 servings per day

List 5—Fats: 8 servings per day

Percentage of calories as carbohydrates: 67

Percentage of calories as fats: 18

Percentage of calories as protein: 15

Protein content: 79 g

Dietary fiber content: 48.5–101.5 g

2,000-CALORIE OMNIVORE DIET

List 1—Vegetables: 5 servings per day

List 2—Fruits: 2.5 servings per day

List 3—Breads, cereals, and starchy vegetables: 13
     servings per day
List 4—Legumes: 2 servings per day
List 5—Fats: 7 servings per day
List 6—Milk: 1 serving per day
List 7—Meats, fish, cheese, and eggs: 2 servings per day

Percentage of calories as carbohydrates: 66
Percentage of calories as fats: 19
Percentage of calories as protein: 15
Protein content: 78 g (72% from plant sources)
Dietary fiber content: 32.5–88.5 g

2,500-CALORIE VEGAN DIET

List 1—Vegetables: 8 servings per day
List 2—Fruits: 3 servings per day
List 3—Breads, cereals, and starchy vegetables: 17
     servings per day
List 4—Legumes: 5 servings per day
List 5—Fats: 8 servings per day

Percentage of calories as carbohydrates: 69
Percentage of calories as fats: 15
Percentage of calories as protein: 16
Protein content: 101 g
Dietary fiber content: 33–121 g

2,500-CALORIE OMNIVORE DIET:

List 1—Vegetables: 8 servings per day

List 2—Fruits: 3.5 servings per day

List 3—Breads, cereals, and starchy vegetables: 17
servings per day

List 4—Legumes: 2 servings per day

List 5—Fats: 8 servings per day

List 6—Milk: 1 serving per day

List 7—Meats, fish, cheese, and eggs: 3 servings per day

Percentage of calories as carbohydrates: 66

Percentage of calories as fats: 18

Percentage of calories as protein: 16

Protein content: 102 g (80% from plant sources)

Dietary fiber content: 40.5–116.5 g

3,000-CALORIE VEGAN DIET:

List 1—Vegetables: 10 servings per day

List 2—Fruits: 4 servings per day

List 3—Breads, cereals, and starchy vegetables: 17
servings per day

List 4—Legumes: 6 servings per day

List 5—Fats: 10 servings per day

Percentage of calories as carbohydrates: 70

Percentage of calories as fats: 16

Percentage of calories as protein: 14
Protein content: 116 g
Dietary fiber content: 50–84 g

3,000-CALORIE OMNIVORE DIET:

List 1—Vegetables: 10 servings per day
List 2—Fruits: 3 servings per day
List 3—Breads, cereals, and starchy vegetables: 20
    servings per day
List 4—Legumes: 2 servings per day
List 5—Fats: 10 servings per day
List 6—Milk: 1 serving per day
List 7—Meats, fish, cheese, and eggs: 3 servings per day

Percentage of calories as carbohydrates: 67
Percentage of calories as fats: 18
Percentage of calories as protein: 15
Protein content: 116 g (81% from plant sources)
Dietary fiber content: 45–133 g

(Note: Use these recommendations as the basis for calculating other calorie diets. For example, for a 4,000-calorie diet add the 2,500 to the 1,500. For a 1,000-calorie diet divide the 2,000-calorie diet in half.)

The Healthy Exchange Lists

EXCHANGE LIST I—VEGETABLES

Vegetables provide the broadest range of nutrients of any food class. They are rich sources of vitamins, minerals, carbohydrates, and protein. The little fat they contain is in the form of essential fatty acids. Vegetables provide high quantities of other valuable health-promoting substances, especially fiber and carotenes. In Latin the word for *vegetable* means "to enliven or animate." Vegetables give us life. More and more evidence is accumulating that shows vegetables can prevent as well as treat many diseases.

Vegetables are the richest sources of antioxidant compounds, which provide protection against free radicals. Free radicals are highly reactive molecules that can bind with and destroy body structures. Free radicals have also been shown to be responsible for the initiation of many diseases, including America's two biggest killers—heart disease and cancer.

The best way to consume many vegetables is in their fresh, raw form. When fresh, many of the nutrients and health-promoting compounds of vegetables are provided in much higher concentrations. If you are going to cook vegetables, it is very important that they not be overcooked. Overcooking will result in a loss of important nutrients. The best ways to cook vegetables are light steaming, baking, grilling and quick stir-frying. Do not boil vegetables unless you are making soup, as much of the nutrients would be left in the water. If fresh vegetables are not available, frozen vegetables are preferred over their canned counterparts.

GRILLED VEGETABLES WITH TARRAGON
(MAKES 6 SERVINGS)

Zucchini, summer squash, eggplant, and bell peppers all benefit from tarragon's anise zing.

4 small to medium zucchini (about 1 pound), cut into
⅓-inch slices

4 small to medium yellow summer squash (about 1 pound), cut into ⅓-inch slices

1 large eggplant, cut crosswise into ⅓-inch slices

2 red bell peppers, cored, seeded, and quartered

4 scallions, cleaned but roots left on

2 tablespoons olive oil

2 tablespoons balsamic vinegar

1 teaspoon Dijon mustard

¼ cup fresh tarragon leaves

Pinch of sea salt

COMBINE the zucchini, squash, eggplant, peppers, and scallions in a large bowl.

IN a small bowl, whisk together the oil, vinegar, mustard, tarragon, and salt. Pour the dressing over the vegetables and toss well. Let the vegetables marinate for at least an hour, or as long as overnight.

PREPARE the grill or preheat the broiler.

USING tongs, lift the vegetables out of the marinade, knocking off the tarragon leaves so that they won't burn. Grill the vegetables 4 inches from the heat, turning once, until cooked through, about 10 to 15 minutes. Remove the individual vegetables as they finish cooking and set them back in the marinade. Serve warm as a light entrée, along with chilled soup, or as an appetizer or side dish.

Exchanges per serving:

Vegetables—1

Fats—1

Marinated vegetables, such as those in the recipe above are healthy choices, but pickled vegetables may not be. Pickled vegetables are not only high in salt, they may also be high in cancer-causing compounds. Several population studies in China have suggested an association between consumption of pickled vegetables and cancer of the esophagus.[7] Pickled vegetables are usually not only high in salt, but also contain high concentrations of N-nitroso compounds. Once ingested, these compounds can form potent cancer-causing nitrosamines.

Vegetables are fantastic "diet" foods, as they are very high in nutritional value but low in calories. In the list below you will notice there is also a list of "free" vegetables. These vegetables are termed free foods and can be eaten in any desired amount because the calories they contain are offset by the number of calories your body burns in the process of digesting them. If you are trying to lose weight, these foods are especially valuable, as they help to keep you feeling satisfied between meals.

The list below shows the vegetables to use for 1 vegetable exchange. One cup cooked vegetables or fresh vegetable juice, or two cups raw vegetables, equals one exchange. Please notice that starchy vegetables such as potatoes and yams are included in the List 3—Breads, cereals, and starchy vegetables.

Artichoke (1 medium)	Mustard
Asparagus	Spinach
Bean sprouts	Turnip
Beets	Mushrooms
Broccoli	Okra
Brussels sprouts	Onions
Carrots	Rhubarb
Cauliflower	Rutabaga
Eggplant	Sauerkraut
Greens:	String beans, green or yellow
Beet	Summer squash
Chard	Tomatoes, tomato juice,
Collard	vegetable juice cocktail
Dandelion	Zucchini
Kale	

The following vegetables may be used as often as desired, especially in their raw form:

Alfalfa sprouts	Cucumber
Bell peppers	Endive
Bok choy	Escarole
Cabbage	Lettuce
Celery	Parsley
Chicory	Radishes
Chinese cabbage	Watercress

EXCHANGE LIST 2—FRUITS

As mentioned previously, fruits are a rich source of many beneficial compounds, and regular fruit consumption has been shown to offer significant protection against many chronic degenerative diseases including cancer, heart disease, cataracts, and strokes. Fruit makes an excellent snack, as it contains fructose or fruit sugar. This sugar is absorbed slowly into the bloodstream, allowing the body time to utilize it. Fruits are also excellent sources of vitamins and minerals as well as health-promoting fiber compounds. However, fruits are not as nutrient dense as vegetables because they are typically higher in calories. That is why vegetables are favored over fruits in weight loss plans and overall healthy diets.

Each of the following equals one exchange:

Fresh juice	1 cup (8 oz.)
Pasteurized juice	⅔ cup
Apple	1 large
Applesauce (unsweetened)	1 cup
Apricots, dried	8 halves

Apricots, fresh	4 medium
Banana	1 medium ✓
Berries	
Blackberries	1 cup
Blueberries	1 cup
Cranberries	1 cup
Raspberries	1 cup
Strawberries	1½ cups
Cherries	20 large
Dates	4
Figs, fresh or dried	2
Grapefruit	1
Grapes	20
Mango	1 small
Melons	
Cantaloupe	½ small
Honeydew	¼ medium
Watermelon	2 cups
Nectarine	2 small
Orange	1 large
Papaya	1½ cups
Peach	2 medium
Persimmon, native	2 medium
Pineapple	1 cup
Plums	4 medium
Prune juice	½ cup
Prunes	4 medium

Raisins	4 tablespoons
Tangerine	2 medium

Additional fruit exchanges: (no more than one per day)

Honey	1 tablespoon
Jams, jellies, preserves	1 tablespoon
Sugar	1 tablespoon

EXCHANGE LIST 3—BREADS, CEREALS, AND STARCHY VEGETABLES

Breads, cereals, and starchy vegetables are classified as complex carbohydrates. Chemically complex carbohydrates are made up of long chains of simple carbohydrates or sugars. This means the body has to digest or break down the large sugar chains into simple sugars. Therefore the sugar from complex carbohydrates enters the bloodstream more slowly. This means blood sugar levels and appetite are better controlled.

Complex carbohydrate foods such as breads, cereals, and starchy vegetables are higher in fiber and nutrients but lower in calories than foods high in simple sugars, such as cakes and candies. Choose whole-grain products (e.g., whole-grain breads, whole-grain flour products, brown rice, etc.) over their processed counterparts (white bread, white flour products, white rice, etc.). Whole grains provide substantially more nutrients and health-promoting properties. Whole grains are a major source of complex carbohydrates, dietary fiber, minerals, and B vitamins. The protein content and quality of whole grains is greater than that of refined grains. Diets rich in whole grains have been shown to be protective against the development of chronic degenerative diseases, especially cancer, heart disease, diabetes, varicose veins, and diseases of the colon including colon cancer, inflammatory bowel disease, hemorrhoids, and diverticulitis.[8]

Whole grains can be used as breakfast cereals, side dishes, casseroles, or used as part of the main entrée. Whole grains are very easy to prepare: Simply rinse the grain to remove any debris; bring the water to boil in an appropriately sized saucepan; stir in the grain; reduce the heat and simmer, covered, for the suggested cooking time; and test for doneness.

Grain (l cup dry)	Water (cups)	Cooking time	Yield (cups)
Barley	3	1¼ hours	3½
Brown rice	2	45 minutes	3
Buckwheat (kasha)	2	15 minutes	2½
Bulgur wheat	2	15–20 minutes	2½
Cornmeal (polenta)	4	25 minutes	3
Cracked wheat	2	25 minutes	2⅓
Millet	3	45 minutes	3½
Quinoa	2¼	20 minutes	2
Whole wheat berries	3	2 hours	2⅔
Wild rice	3	1 hour	4

Potatoes and other starchy vegetables are also quite versatile. Here is a recipe for a delicious potato salad:

BAKED POTATO SALAD WITH
FRESH CHERVIL

(MAKES 6 SERVINGS)

Chervil and mustard combine to give baked potatoes a rich flavor without adding any fat.

3 pounds baking potatoes (about 3 large ones)

3 scallions, minced

2 tablespoons very finely minced red onion

½ cup plain nonfat yogurt

2 teaspoons coarse mustard

2 tablespoons minced fresh chervil

PREHEAT the oven to 500°F.

RINSE the potatoes and poke each in about five places with a knife. Bake, right on the oven rack, until just tender, 45 to 60 minutes, depending on the variety of potato.

MEANWHILE, in a large bowl, combine the scallions, onion, yogurt, mustard, and chervil.

LET the potatoes cool on a wire cake rack, to keep them from getting soggy, until they're cool enough to handle. Cut them into slices and add to the yogurt mixture. Combine gently with a rubber spatula so that the slices don't crumble; it's okay if a few break. Serve warm or very slightly chilled.

Exchanges per serving:
Breads, Cereals, and Starchy Vegetables—1

One of the following equals one exchange:

Breads
Bagel	1
Dinner roll	1
Dried bread crumbs	3 tablespoons
English muffin, small	½
Tortilla (6 inch)	1
Whole wheat, rye, or pumpernickel	1 slice

Cereals
Bran flakes	½ cup
Cereal (cooked)	½ cup
Cornmeal (dry)	2 tablespoons
Flour	2½ tablespoons
Grits (cooked)	½ cup
Pasta (cooked)	½ cup
Puffed cereal (unsweetened)	1 cup
Rice or barley (cooked)	½ cup
Wheat germ	¼ cup
Other unsweetened cereal	¾ cup

Crackers

Arrowroot	3
Graham (2½" square)	2
Matzo (4" × 6")	½
Rye wafers (2" × 3½")	3
Saltines	6

Starchy vegetables

Corn	⅓ cup
Corn on the cob	1 small
Parsnips	⅔ cup
Potato, mashed	½ cup
Potato, white	1 small
Squash, winter, acorn, or butternut	½ cup
Yam or sweet potato	¼ cup

Prepared foods

Biscuit, 2" diameter (plus 1 fat exchange)	1
Corn bread, 2" × 2" × 1" (plus 1 fat exchange)	1
French fries, 2"–3" long (plus 1 fat exchange)	8
Muffin, small (plus 1 fat exchange)	1
Pancake, 5" × ½" (plus 1 fat exchange)	1
Potato or corn chips (plus 2 fat exchanges)	15
Waffle, 5" × ½" (plus 1 fat exchange)	1

EXCHANGE LIST 4—LEGUMES

Legumes (beans) are among the oldest of cultivated plants. Fossil records demonstrate that even prehistoric people domesticated and cultivated certain legumes for food. Today legumes are a mainstay in most diets of the world. Legumes are second only to grains in supplying calories and protein to the world's population. Compared with grains, they supply about the same number of total calories, but usually provide two to four times as much protein.

Legumes are often called the poor people's meat; however, they might be better known as the healthy people's meat. Although legumes lack some key amino acids, when combined with grains they form what is known as a complete protein. Here is one of my favorite high-protein vegetarian meals from my book *The Healing Power of Foods:*

BLACK-EYED PEAS AND BROWN RICE

(MAKES 6 SERVINGS)

1 cup dried black-eyed peas, picked over, rinsed, soaked 10 hours or longer in water
     to cover by at least 4 inches, and drained

5 cups water, divided

¾ teaspoon sea salt, divided

1 cup basmati rice or long-grain brown rice

1 tablespoon canola oil or olive oil

1½ cups finely chopped onions

2 large cloves garlic, peeled and minced

1 tablespoon grated or minced ginger (optional)

1 tablespoon diced green chili or jalapeño, fresh or canned, seeded (optional)

1 teaspoon molasses

IN a medium-size saucepan, cook the peas in 3 cups of the water for 40 minutes. Add ½ teaspoon of the salt (if desired), and cook the peas for another 20 minutes, or until they are tender. Drain the peas, saving ¼ cup of the cooking liquid. Set the peas and the reserved cooking liquid aside.

MEANWHILE, in another medium-size saucepan, combine the rice and the remaining 2 cups of water. Bring the rice to a boil, reduce the heat to low, cover the saucepan, and simmer the rice for 35 to 40 minutes. When the water is fully absorbed and the rice tender, turn off the heat, letting the pan sit, covered, on the stove.

AFTER the peas and rice have cooked for 15 minutes, in a large, heavy skillet, preferably one with a nonstick surface, heat the oil, add the onions, garlic, ginger, and chili or jalapeño, and sauté the vegetables over medium-high heat for 5 minutes. Reduce the heat to medium-low, add the peas, the remaining ¼ teaspoon of salt (if desired), the molasses, and, if needed, more liquid. Cook the mixture, stirring it, for 20 minutes. Serve the peas with the cooked rice.

Exchanges per serving:

Vegetables—⅙

Fruits—⅙

Breads, cereals, and starchy vegetables—⅓
Legumes—⅓

Legumes are fantastic foods, as they are rich in important nutrients and health-promoting compounds. Legumes help improve liver function. lower cholesterol levels, and are extremely effective in improving blood sugar control.[9] Since obesity and diabetes has been linked to loss of blood sugar control due to insulin insensitivity, legumes appear to be extremely important in weight loss plans and diabetes.

Dried legumes are best prepared by first rinsing them to remove any debris and then soaking them overnight in an appropriate amount of water (see below). This is best done in the refrigerator to prevent fermentation. Soaking will usually cut the cooking time dramatically. To check to see if the legume is done, simply let a few cool and taste them. They should be firm but not crunchy. Also look to see if some of the beans have split skins; too many split skins may indicate that the legume has been overcooked. If soaking overnight is not possible, here is an alternate method: Place the dried legumes in an appropriate amount of water in a pot, for each cup of dried legumes add ¼ teaspoon of baking soda, bring to boil for at least 2 minutes, and then set aside to soak for at least an hour. The baking soda will soften the legumes and help break down the troublesome oligosaccharides, which can cause flatulence. The baking soda will also help reduce the amount of cooking time. After soaking, beans should be simmered with a minimum of stirring to keep them firm and unbroken. A pressure cooker or Crock-Pot can also be used for convenience.

Legume (I cup dry)	Water (cups)	Cooking time (hours)	Yield (cups)
Baby limas	2	1½	1¾
Black beans	4	1½	2
Black-eyed peas	3	1	2
Garbanzos (chick-peas)	2	3	2
Great northern beans	3½	2	2
Kidney beans	3	1½	2
Lentils and split peas	3	1	2¼
Limas	2	1½	1¼
Pinto beans	3	2½	2
Red beans	3	3	2
Small white beans (navy)	2	1½	2
Soybeans	3	3	2

The soybean is the most widely grown and utilized legume. It accounts for well over 50 percent of the world's total legume production. In terms of dollar value the soybean is the United States' most important crop, ranking above corn, wheat, and cotton. Unfortunately, in our country, despite its use in a variety of food products, the soybean is still used primarily for animal feed (protein meal) as well as for its oil. However, since the 1970s there has been a marked increase in both the consumption of traditional soyfoods, such as tofu, tempeh, and miso, and in the development of so-called second-generation soyfoods, which simulate traditional meat and dairy products. Consumers can now find soy milk, soy hot dogs, soy sausage, soy cheese, and soy frozen desserts at their grocery stores. One serving (as listed on the package) of a second-generation soyfood equals one exchange.

The increase in soyfood consumption is attributed to a number of factors, including economics, health benefits, and environmental concerns. In terms of cost, soybeans provide a great amount of nutrition per acre. In fact an acre of soybeans can provide nearly twenty times the amount of protein of an acre used for raising beef. Soy consumption is also linked to a reduced risk of cancer and heart disease.

One-half cup of the following cooked or sprouted beans equals one exchange:

Black-eyed peas	Pinto Beans
Chick-peas	Soybeans, including tofu
Garbanzo beans	(plus 1 fat exchange)
Kidney beans	Split peas
Lentils	Other dried beans and peas
Lima Beans	

EXCHANGE LIST 5: FATS AND OILS

Our bodies require certain oils, specifically linoleic and linolenic acid, which are essential to our body's functioning. These polyunsaturated fatty acids function in our bodies as components of nerve cells, cellular membranes, and hormonelike substances known as prostaglandins. Increased consumption of essential fatty acids has been shown to lower cholesterol levels.

When organizations such as the American Cancer Society and the American Heart Association recommend that the diet contain less than 30 percent of calories as fat, what they are really talking about is reducing the amount of "nonessential fats," such as saturated fats, margarine, and partially hydrogenated oils. These same groups also recommend that at least twice as much polyunsaturated fats be consumed as saturated fats.

Saturated fats are typically animal fats and are solid at room temperature. There is a great deal of research linking a diet high in saturated fat to numerous cancers, heart disease, and strokes. Saturated fats are also known to exert negative effects on glucose control by reducing the sensitivity of cells to insulin. As a result, a high intake of saturated fat can result in obesity.

Even more deadly than saturated fats are the trans-fatty acids and partially hydrogenated oils found in margarine and most processed foods. These fats have been implicated as contributing to the following disorders:

- Increased incidence of obesity
- Increased susceptibility to diabetes
- Increased incidence of heart disease
- Increased levels of harmful cholesterol levels in humans

- Increased risk for cancer
- Low birth-weight infants
- Low quality and volume of breast milk
- Abnormal sperm production
- Increased incidence of prostate disease
- Immune suppression
- Essential fatty acid deficiencies

Many researchers and nutritionists have been concerned about the health effects of margarine since it was first introduced. Although many Americans assume they are doing their body good by consuming margarine versus butter and saturated fats, in truth they are actually doing more harm. Margarine and other hydrogenated vegetable oils not only raise LDL cholesterol, they also lower the protective HDL cholesterol level, interfere with essential fatty acid metabolism, and are suspected of being causes of certain cancers.[9] Although butter may be better than margarine, the bottom line is that they both need to be restricted in a healthy diet.

While too much fat is obviously a problem, so is an insufficiency of essential fatty acids. The best recommendation is easy to follow: Simply reduce the amount of animal products in the diet (source of saturated fats) and increase the amount of vegetables, legumes, nuts, and seeds consumed. In addition I would recommend supplementing the diet with a high-quality flaxseed oil. One tablespoon of flaxseed oil per day (3 fat exchanges) is recommended. In addition to flaxseed oil, omega-3 fatty acids are found in cold-water fish (salmon, mackerel, herring, etc.).

The reason I recommend flaxseed oil to most of my patients is that it is nature's richest source of alpha-linolenic acid, the essential omega-3 fatty acid. Omega-3 fatty acids have been shown to improve insulin action, while an excess of saturated fat and a relative insufficiency of essential fatty acids is linked to insulin insensitivity and type II diabetes.[10]

The key reason for these associations of the type of fats consumed and insulin sensitivity is due to the effect of dietary fats on cell membrane fluidity. According to modern pathology, or the study of disease processes, an alteration in cell membrane function is the central factor in the development of cell injury and death.[11] Without a healthy membrane cells lose their ability to hold water, vital nutrients, and electrolytes. They also lose their ability to communicate with other cells and be controlled by regulating hormones. They simply do not function properly. Loss of proper membrane fluidity due to lack of omega-3 fatty acids and too much saturated fat may be the most important reason for insulin insensitivity in many overweight individuals and type II diabetics.[11]

Population studies have shown that frequent consumption of a small amount of omega-3 oils protects against the development of type II diabetes.[12] In addition animal studies have also shown that omega-3 fatty acids prevent the development of insulin resistance.[13] All of this evidence appears to indicate that altered membrane fluidity may play a critical role in the development of not only type II diabetes but also obesity.

To better determine the role of specific fatty acids in increasing the risk of developing type II diabetes, researchers recently examined the fatty-acid composition in the blood among fifty-year-old men in a ten-year follow-up to the famous Uppsala study.[14] The researchers analyzed the blood for a special type of marker (the fatty-acid composition of the serum cholesterol esters) that reflects the average quality of fat consumed over several weeks or perhaps even longer periods of time. Of the 1,828 men who did not have diabetes in 1970–1973, 75 developed type II diabetes.

The results of the study showed striking differences between the two groups. The subjects with diabetes had higher proportions of saturated fatty acids and a fatty-acid pattern that is associated with a high intake of meat and dairy products along with a low intake of vegetable oils.

The results of this study indicate the following dietary recommendations related to fatty-acid intake might significantly improve insulin sensitivity and reduce the risk of developing type II diabetes:

- Reduce the intake of saturated fatty acids
- Increase the consumption of essential fatty acids (linoleic and alpha-linolenic acids)
- Increase consumption of omega-3 oils by consuming cold-water fish and/or flaxseed oil

One of the best ways to incorporate flaxseed oil into the diet is to use it to make your own salad dressings. Most commercially available salad dressings, as well as those in restaurants, are full of the wrong type of fats and oils. You can also use medium-chain triglycerides, a special type of fat with weight-loss-promoting effects that is discussed in chapter 7. Here is a recipe for making your own salad dressing from my book *The Healing Power of Foods*:

BASIL DRESSING

(MAKES 12 ONE-TABLESPOON SERVINGS)

¼ cup flaxseed oil or medium-chain triglycerides

3 tablespoons fresh lemon juice

¼ cup water

2 tablespoons minced fresh basil or 1½ teaspoons dried basil

1 teaspoon finely chopped garlic

Black pepper to taste

COMBINE all ingredients in a blender or food processor and mix thoroughly.

If you would like other flaxseed oil recipes, contact Barlean's Organic Oils (1-800-445-3529). There is also an excellent recipe book entitled *Flax for Life—101 Delicious Recipes and Tips Featuring Flaxseed Oil*, by Jade Beutler.

Another way of increasing the intake of essential fatty acids is increasing the consumption of nuts and seeds. Nuts and seeds provide excellent nutrition. They are especially good sources of essential fatty acids, vitamin E, protein, minerals, fiber and other health-promoting substances.

Because nuts and seeds have a high oil content, one would suspect that frequent consumption of nuts would increase the rate of obesity. But in a large population study of 26,473 Americans it was found that people who consumed the most nuts were less obese than those who consumed few. This statistic is quite interesting and may reflect improved insulin sensitivity and dietary thermogenesis. Another possible explanation is that the nuts produced satiety, a feeling of appetite satisfaction. This same study also demonstrated that higher nut consumption was associated with a protective effect against heart attacks (both fatal and nonfatal).[15]

Results in a recent study designed to better understand the beneficial effects of nuts against heart disease published in the prestigious *New England Journal of Medicine* show that walnut consumption lowered total cholesterol 12.4 percent, reduced LDL-cholesterol 16.3 percent, and decreased triglyceride levels 8.3 percent in men with normal blood cholesterol and triglyceride levels.[16] Although this study utilized walnuts, presumably other nuts exert similar effects on blood cholesterol and triglyceride levels. The beneficial effects are thought to be due to the essential fatty acids, especially the omega-3 fatty acid alpha-linolenic acid.

In general, nuts and seeds, due to their high oil content, are best purchased and stored in their shells. The shell is a natural protector against free-radical damage caused by light and air. Make sure the shells are free of splits, cracks, stains, holes, or other surface imperfections. Do not eat or use moldy nuts or seeds, as this may not be safe. Also avoid limp, rubbery, dark, or shriveled nut meats. Store nuts and seeds with shells in a cool, dry place. If whole nuts and seeds with their shells are not available, make sure they are stored in airtight containers in the refrigerator or freezer. Crushed nuts, slivered nuts, and nut pieces can often be rancid. Prepare your own from the whole nut if a recipe calls for these.

Each of the following equals one exchange:

Polyunsaturated:
    Vegetable oils: 1 teaspoon
        Canola
        Corn
        Flax
        Safflower
        Soy
        Sunflower
    Avocado (4" diameter)   ⅛
    Almonds   10 whole
    Peanuts:
        Spanish   20 whole
        Virginia   10 whole
    Pecans   2 large
    Seeds: 1 tablespoon
        Flax
        Pumpkin

Sesame

Sunflower

Walnuts   6 small

Mono-unsaturated:

    Olive oil   1 teaspoon

    Olives   5 small

Saturated: (avoid)

    Bacon   1 slice

    Butter   1 teaspoon

    Cream, heavy   1 tablespoon

    Cream, light or sour   2 tablespoons

    Cream cheese   1 tablespoon

    Mayonnaise   1 teaspoon

    Salad dressings   2 teaspoons

EXCHANGE LIST 6—MILK

Is milk for "everybody"? Definitely not. Many people are allergic to milk or lack the necessary enzymes to digest milk. Another reason to avoid milk is that a milk protein known as casein may promote atherosclerosis.[17] Many meal replacement formulas, including Ultra SlimFast, contain casein. Casein is also used in glues, molded plastics, and paints. A good alternative to milk and casein-containing formulas is using soy milk or soy-based formulas. Unlike casein, soy protein actually lowers cholesterol levels.[18]

Certainly milk consumption should be limited to no more than one or two servings per day. Choose nonfat products.

One cup equals one exchange:

Nonfat milk or yogurt
2% milk (plus 1 fat exchange)
Low-fat yogurt (plus 1 fat exchange)
Low-fat cottage cheese (plus 1 fat exchange)
Whole milk (plus 2 fat exchanges)
Whole-milk yogurt (plus 2 fat exchanges)

EXCHANGE LIST 7: MEATS, FISH, CHEESE, AND EGGS

When choosing from this list, it is important to choose primarily from the low-fat group and remove the skin of poultry. This will keep the amount of saturated fat low. Although many people advocate vegetarianism, the exchange list below provides high concentrations of certain nutrients difficult to get in an entirely vegetarian diet, such as the full range of amino acids, vitamin B_{12}, and iron. The most important recommendation may be to use these foods in small amounts as "condiments" in the diet rather than as the mainstay.

Each of the following equals one exchange:

Low fat (less than 15% fat content):

Beef: baby beef, chipped beef, chuck, steak (flank, plate), tenderloin plate ribs, round (bottom, top), all cuts rump, spareribs	1 ounce
Fish	1 ounce
Lamb: leg, rib, sirloin, loin (roast and chops), shank, shoulder	1 ounce
Poultry: chicken or turkey without skin	1 ounce
Veal: leg, loin, rib, shank, shoulder, cutlet	1 ounce

Medium fat (for each selection add ½ fat exchange):

Beef: ground (15% fat), canned corned beef, rib eye, round (ground commercial)	1 ounce
Cheese: mozzarella, ricotta, Parmesan	1 ounce
Eggs	1
Organ meats	1 ounce
Peanut butter	2 tablespoons
Pork: loin (all tenderloin), picnic and boiled ham, shoulder, Canadian bacon	1 ounce

High fat (for each exchange plus 1 fat exchange):

Beef: brisket, corned beef, ground beef (more than 20% fat), hamburger, roasts (rib), steaks (club and rib)	1 ounce
Cheese, Cheddar	1 ounce
Duck or goose	1 ounce
Lamb: breast	1 ounce
Pork: spareribs, loin, ground pork, country-style ham, deviled ham	1 ounce

The Importance of Menu Planning

When trying to eat for health, it is very important to spend time planning out daily menus in advance. The Healthy Exchange System was created to ensure that you consume a healthy diet that provides adequate levels of nutrients in the proper ratio. It is important to determine your desired calorie intake and to calculate the number of servings required from each Healthy Exchange List. This will help a great deal when constructing a daily menu.

The recipes provided in this book have incorporated the Healthy Exchange System. If you would like a good cookbook that also incorporates the Healthy Exchange System, please get my *Healing Power of Foods Cookbook*. If you cannot find it in your local health food store or bookstore, call 1-800-477-2995.

BREAKFAST

Do not skip breakfast. The best foods to eat for breakfast are cereals, both hot and cold, and preferably from whole grains without added fat, sugar, or salt. Instead of using cow's milk, try soy milk (note: I like Westsoy Lite and Pacific Foods Ultra Soy Beverage, vanilla-flavored). Cereals are the best choice for breakfast because data from the National Health and Nutrition Examination Survey II (a national survey of the nutritional and health practices of Americans) disclosed that serum cholesterol levels are lowest among adults eating whole-grain cereal for breakfast.[19] Although those individuals who consumed other breakfast foods had higher blood cholesterol levels, levels were highest among those who typically skipped breakfast.

The table opposite lists the calorie and fiber content of several cereals. The best choices are All-Bran, Shredded Wheat, oatmeal, and Bran Chex. Although Shredded Wheat and oatmeal may not be as high in fiber as the "bran" cereals, the serving size is larger and they tend to be more satisfying to the appetite. Cornflakes and Grape-Nuts are poor choices—Grape-Nuts because the serving size is small and the level of fiber is on the low end, and cornflakes because of the low fiber content. Also avoid granola-type cold cereals, as they tend to be full of extra calories due to the addition of oil and sugar.

Calorie and Fiber Content of Selected Cereals

Cereal	Serving size	Calories	Grams of fiber
All–Bran	⅓ cup	71	8.5
Bran Chex	⅔ cup	91	4.6
Corn Bran	⅔ cup	98	5.4
Cornflakes	1¼ cup	110	0.3
Grape-Nuts	¼ cup	101	1.4
Oatmeal	¾ cup	108	1.6
Raisin Bran–type	⅔ cup	115	4.0
Shredded Wheat	⅔ cup	102	2.6

LUNCH

Lunch is a great time to enjoy a healthy bowl of soup and a large salad. Bean soups and other legume dishes are especially good lunch selections for people with diabetes and blood sugar problems due to their ability to improve blood sugar regulation. Legumes are filling yet low in calories.

Calorie and Fiber Content of Legumes

Legume	Serving size	Calories	Grams of fiber
Dried peas, cooked	½ cup	115	4.7
Kidney beans, cooked	½ cup	110	7.3
Lentils, cooked	½ cup	97	3.7

Lima beans, cooked	½ cup	64	4.5
Navy beans, cooked	½ cup	112	6.0

Here are two recipes for delicious, health-promoting, and appetite-satisfying salads that make an excellent lunch.

CHICK-PEA SALAD WITH RED ONION AND MUSTARD GREENS
(MAKES 2 SERVINGS)

1 tablespoon fresh lemon juice

1 tablespoon red wine vinegar

2 teaspoons olive or flaxseed oil

½ teaspoon Dijon mustard

1 clove garlic, mashed through a press

1 teaspoon minced fresh oregano or ½ teaspoon dried

2 cups cooked chick-peas (canned are okay, but rinse before using)

1½ cups thinly sliced mustard greens

1 small red onion, thinly sliced and separated into rings

IN a small bowl, whisk together the lemon juice, vinegar, oil, and mustard. Stir in the garlic and oregano.

PUT the chick-peas, mustard greens, and onion into a medium bowl. Add the dressing, and toss well to coat. Serve at room temperature or very slightly chilled as a side dish or appetizer.

Exchanges per serving:

Vegetables—1

Legumes—2

WHITE BEAN SALAD WITH LEMON AND DILL

(MAKES 2 SERVINGS)

2 cups cooked white beans (if using canned beans, rinse, drain, and pat dry)

1 cup cooked tiny pasta, such as orzo, elbow macaroni, or ditalini (from about 2
     ounces dried)

⅓ cup finely minced celery

⅓ cup finely minced red bell pepper

3 scallions, finely minced

Juice of ½ lemon

1 teaspoon olive oil

1 clove garlic, very finely minced

1 teaspoon minced fresh dill

Curly red lettuce or purple perilla for serving

COMBINE the beans, pasta, celery, bell pepper, and scallions in a large bowl.

IN a small bowl, whisk together the lemon juice, olive oil, garlic, and dill. Pour over the bean mixture and toss well to combine. Serve at room temperature or very slightly chilled on a nest of red lettuce, for lunch or a light dinner.

Exchanges per serving:

Breads, cereals, and starchy vegetables—¼

Legumes—2

SNACKS

The best snacks are fresh fruits and vegetables. Fresh apple, pear, and grapefruit are high in pectin, a very good water-soluble fiber useful as a weight loss aid (see page 121). Vegetable sticks are also good snacks. If you find you are quite hungry, here is a great tip: Always have handy a couple of rye crispbread crackers (Wasa and Ryvita are good brands). When hungry, eat one or two crackers and drink a large glass of water. The rye fiber in the cracker will expand in the water to produce a feeling of fullness in the stomach. You can also take a fiber supplement (discussed in chapter 7) to produce the same effect without the calories of the cracker. Raw nuts and seeds are also good snack choices.

Calorie and Fiber Content of Selected Raw Fruits and Vegetables

Fruit	Serving size	Calories	Grams of fiber
Apple (with skin)	1 medium	81	3.5
Banana	1 medium	105	2.4
Cantaloupe	¼ melon	30	1.0
Cherries, sweet	10	49	1.2
Grapefruit	½ medium	38	1.6
Orange	1 medium	62	2.6
Peach (with skin)	1	37	1.9

Pear (with skin)	½ large	61	3.1
Prunes	3	60	3.0
Raisins	¼ cup	106	3.1
Raspberries	½ cup	35	3.1
Strawberries	1 cup	45	3.0

Vegetable	Serving size	Calories	Grams of fiber
Bean sprouts	1 cup	26	3.0
Celery, diced	1 cup	20	2.2
Cucumber	1 cup	16	0.8
Lettuce	1 cup	20	1.8
Mushrooms	1 cup	20	3.0
Pepper, green	1 cup	18	1.0
Spinach	1 cup	16	2.4
Tomato	1 medium	20	1.5

Note: If you were to have all the vegetables in the table above as a salad, it would provide 7 cups of food and 15.7 grams of fiber, and yet only have 156 calories!

DINNER

For dinner the healthiest meals contain a fresh vegetable salad, a cooked vegetable side dish or a bowl of soup, whole grains, and legumes. The whole grains may be provided in bread, pasta, or as a side dish or part of a recipe for an entrée. The legumes can be utilized in soups, salads, and main entrées. As an example, one of my favorite meals is Insalata Mista Salad, a whole-grain roll, and Polenta Puttanesca (recipes follow).

INSALATA MISTA SALAD

(MAKES 4 SERVINGS)

1 head of lettuce

1 fennel bulb

½ small cucumber, sliced

6 radishes, trimmed and sliced

1 celery heart, chopped

1 small green pepper, cored, deseeded, and sliced

4 scallions, thinly sliced

2 ripe, firm tomatoes

Lite Salt or salt substitute

2 tablespoons olive oil, flaxseed oil, or medium-chain triglycerides

2 teaspoons cider vinegar or lemon juice

PULL off and discard any of the lettuce's bruised or blemished outer leaves. Wash and shake dry in a salad basket. Tear into bite-size pieces and place in a salad bowl. Trim the stalks, base, and coarse outer leaves from the fennel; cut downward into thin slices, then into strips. Add to the salad bowl with the cucumber, radishes, celery, pepper, and scallions. Cut the tomatoes into quarters, then in eighths, and add to the bowl. When ready to serve, sprinkle with a little salt and add the oil and the cider vinegar or lemon juice and toss lightly together. Serve immediately.

Exchanges per serving:

Vegetables—¾

Fats—½

POLENTA PUTTANESCA

(MAKES 4 SERVINGS)

SAUCE

1 tablespoon olive oil

7 cloves garlic

¼ teaspoon dried red pepper flakes

2 large green peppers, cut into strips

2 pounds of tomatoes, chopped and drained

2 tablespoons tomato paste

6 black olives, halved

2 teaspoons capers

¼ teaspoon Lite Salt or salt substitute

Ground pepper

POLENTA

4 cups water

1¼ cups cornmeal

⅓ teaspoon Lite Salt or salt substitute

⅓ cup grated soy cheese

continued

IN a large skillet, heat the oil over medium heat until hot. Then add the garlic and red pepper flakes. Cook for 3 minutes. Add the green peppers and sauté 10 minutes. Add the tomatoes, tomato paste, olives, capers, Lite Salt or salt substitute, and pepper. Cook until the peppers are tender and the sauce thickens.

MEANWHILE make the polenta. In a medium saucepan, bring the water to a boil. Drizzle in the polenta slowly, whisking continuously with a wire whisk all the while it is being sprinkled in. Add the Lite Salt or salt substitute and reduce the heat to low. Continue to whisk polenta until it is a thick mass. Stir continuously until the polenta pulls away from the sides of the pan (5 to 7 minutes)

TO serve, spoon equal portions of the polenta onto the center of each serving plate. Top with the sauce and serve immediately.

Exchanges per serving:
Vegetables—1½
Grains and starches—2
Fats—1
Milk—⅛

Although a mixed, varied diet rich in whole grains, vegetables, and legumes provides optimal levels of protein, some people like to eat meat. The important thing is not to overconsume animal products. Limit your intake to no more than

4 ounces per day and choose fish, skinless poultry, and lean cuts rather than fat-laden choices.

Because of the high allotment for vegetables in the Healthy Exchange System, you will probably find yourself consuming lots of salads and steamed vegetables, which are high in nutritional value and dietary fiber and low in calories. The best choices for steamed vegetables are any vegetables other than the starchy ones (potatoes, sweet potatoes, and parsnips).

Calorie and Fiber Content of Steamed Vegetables

Vegetable	Serving size	Calories	Grams of fiber
Asparagus, cut	1 cup	30	2.0
Beans, green	1 cup	32	3.2
Broccoli	1 cup	40	4.4
Brussels sprouts	1 cup	56	4.6
Cabbage, red	1 cup	30	2.8
Carrots	1 cup	48	4.6
Cauliflower	1 cup	28	2.2
Corn	1 cup	87	2.9
Kale	1 cup	44	2.8
Parsnip	1 cup	102	5.4
Potato (with skin)	1 medium	106	2.5
Potato (without skin)	1 medium	97	1.4
Spinach	1 cup	42	4.2
Sweet potatoes	1 medium	160	3.4
Zucchini	1 cup	22	3.6

Here are a couple of excellent vegetable dishes that I really enjoy:

SPICY EGGPLANT SALAD

(MAKES 4 SERVINGS)

In the cuisines of India, coriander seed is often paired with cumin seed and hot pepper.

1½ pounds eggplant, cut into chunks

3 bay leaves

2 teaspoons olive oil

2 cloves garlic, mashed through a press

1 leek, topped, tailed, rinsed, and minced

1 teaspoon finely grated fresh ginger

1 teaspoon cumin seed, crushed

1 teaspoon coriander seed, crushed

1 dried hot chili pepper (about 1 inch long), crushed, or 1 teaspoon dried hot red pepper flakes

2 medium tomatoes, chopped

1 red bell pepper, cored, seeded, and chopped

2 scallions, minced

2 tablespoons minced coriander leaves

PLACE the eggplant on a steamer rack and steam over boiling water, to which you've added the bay leaves, until very tender, about 10 to 12 minutes.

MEANWHILE, heat a medium sauté pan over medium-high heat. Pour in the oil, then add the garlic, leek, ginger, cumin seed, coriander seed, hot pepper, tomatoes, and bell pepper and sauté until fragrant and saucy, about 4 minutes.

COMBINE the steamed eggplant with the tomato mixture in a shallow bowl, taking care not to squash the eggplant. Sprinkle with the scallions and coriander leaves and serve warm or slightly chilled.

Exchanges per serving:

Vegetables—2

STIR-FRIED VEGETABLES

(MAKES 8 SERVINGS)

I teaspoon canola oil

2 tablespoons minced gingerroot

¼ head cauliflower, separated into florets

¼ pound broccoli, separated into florets

½ cup julienne-cut celery

¼ pound pea pods

¼ head napa cabbage, shredded

10 mushrooms, diced

¼ pound bamboo shoots, diced

I tablespoon low-sodium soy sauce

½ cup thinly sliced water chestnuts

I medium onion, thinly sliced

¼ pound bean sprouts

continued

IN a heated wok or skillet, warm canola oil. Add gingerroot, cauliflower, broccoli, celery, and pea pods. Stir-fry for 2 minutes over high heat. Add cabbage, mushrooms, and bamboo shoots. Stir-fry for 1 minute more. Stir in soy sauce and simmer over low heat for 1 minute. Add water chestnuts, onion, and bean sprouts and stir-fry for 1 minute over high heat until tender-crisp. Stir-frying vegetables is perhaps the quickest way to cook them (microwave excluded). Don't overcook the vegetables, as this will cause loss of much nutritional value.

Exchanges per serving:
Vegetables—I
Fats—I

Final Comments

A diet high in complex carbohydrate and dietary fiber and low in saturated fat is clearly the diet of choice for optimum health and achieving ideal body weight. Although the body should be low in total fat, it is necessary to provide the essential fatty acids. Be sure to consume flaxseed oil and fresh, raw nuts and seeds on a regular basis. The Healthy Exchange System presented in this chapter allows for the construction of a diet that provides flexibility and long-term success.

Chapter 4

The Importance of Exercise

Regular exercise is an absolute must in order to lose weight and keep it off. Despite the fact that everyone agrees that exercise is vital to good health, less than 20 percent of Americans exercise on a regular basis. It is absolutely essential that you overcome in yourself any excuse not to exercise. Create the time, energy, and motivation that you need to make exercise a part of your daily routine. If you kept your dietary intake the same as it is now and simply exercised for 25 to 30 minutes a day at a moderate intensity level, over the course of a year you would lose 20 to 25 pounds. Combining exercise with the dietary guidelines given in the previous chapter will make the pounds come off!

While the immediate effect of exercise is stress on the body, regular exercise causes the body to adapt—it becomes stronger, functions more efficiently, and has greater endurance. The entire body benefits from regular exercise, largely as a result of improved cardiovascular and respiratory function. Simply stated, exercise enhances the transport of oxygen and nutrients into the cells. At the same time exercise enhances the transport of carbon dioxide and waste products from the tissues of the body to the bloodstream and ultimately to the eliminative organs. As a result regular exercise increases stamina and energy levels.

Regular exercise is particularly important in reducing the risk of heart disease. It does this by lowering cholesterol levels, improving blood and oxygen supply to the heart, increasing the functional capacity of the heart, reducing blood pressure, reducing obesity, and exerting a favorable effect on blood clotting.[1]

Exercise and Weight Loss

Physical inactivity is a major reason why so many Americans are overweight. This is especially true in children. Studies have demonstrated that childhood obesity is associated more with inactivity than with overeating.[2] Since strong evidence suggests that 80 to 86 percent of adult obesity begins in childhood, one can conclude that lack of physical activity is a major cause of obesity.

People who tend to be physically active tend to have less of a problem with weight loss. Regular exercise is a necessary component of any effective weight loss program because of the following factors:

- When weight loss is achieved by dieting without exercise, a substantial portion of the total weight loss comes from muscle tissue and water loss.
- When exercise is included in a weight loss program, the percentage of muscle to fat improves. Lean body weight increases because of an increase in muscle mass and a decrease in body fat. Since muscle burns calories, whereas fat stores calories, an increase in muscle mass means your body is burning more calories all day long—even while you're asleep.
- Exercise helps counter the reduction in basal metabolic rate (BMR)—the rate at which your body burns calories when you're inactive or at rest—that usually accompanies dieting alone and is also associated with aging.
- Exercise increases metabolism, not just when you're exercising but for an extended period of time following the exercise session.
- Moderate to intense exercise may have a suppressing effect on the appetite.
- Those subjects who exercise during and after weight reduction are better able to maintain their weight loss than those who do not exercise, presumably due to all of the reasons given above.

Exercise promotes the development of an efficient method of burning fat. Muscle tissue is the primary user of fat calories in the body, so the greater your muscle mass, the greater your fat-burning capacity. If you want to be healthy and achieve your ideal body weight, you must exercise.

Exercise Improves Self-esteem

Regular exercise also exerts a powerful positive effect on the mind and attitude. Tensions, depressions, feelings of inadequacy, and worries diminish greatly with regular exercise. Exercise alone has been demonstrated to have a tremendous impact on improving mood and the ability to handle life's stressful situations.

A study published in the *American Journal of Epidemiology* found that increased participation in exercise, sports, and physical activities is strongly associated with decreased symptoms of anxiety (restlessness, tension, etc.), depression (feelings that life is not worthwhile, low spirits, etc.), and malaise (run-down feeling, insomnia, etc.). Simply stated, people who participate in regular exercise have higher self-esteem, feel better, and are happier.[3]

Regular exercise has also been shown to enhance powerful mood-elevating substances in the brain known as endorphins.[4] These compounds exert effects similar to morphine. In fact their name (*endo* = endogenous, *-rphins* = morphines) was given to them because of their morphinelike effects. A clear association exists between exercise and endorphin elevation, and when endorphins go up, mood follows.

Dennis Lobstein, Ph.D., a professor of exercise psychobiology at the University of New Mexico, compared the beta-endorphin levels and depression profiles of ten joggers versus ten sedentary men of the same age. The ten sedentary men tested out more depressed, perceived greater stress in their lives, and had more stress-circulating hormones and lower levels of beta-endorphins. As Dr. Lobstein stated, this "reaffirms that depression is very sensitive to exercise and helps firm up a biochemical link between physical activity and depression."[5]

Benefits of Exercise

Musculoskeletal System
- Increases muscle strength
- Increases flexibility of muscles and range of joint motion
- Produces stronger bones, ligaments, and tendons
- Lessens chance of injury
- Enhances posture, poise, and physique

Heart and Blood Vessels
- Lowers resting heart rate
- Strengthens heart function
- Lowers blood pressure
- Improves oxygen delivery throughout the body

- Increases blood supply to muscles
- Enlarges the arteries to the heart

Bodily Processes
- Reduces heart disease risk
- Helps lower blood cholesterol and triglycerides
- Raises HDL, the "good" cholesterol
- Helps improve calcium deposition in bones
- Prevents osteoporosis
- Improves immune function
- Aids digestion
- Increases lean body mass
- Improves the body's ability to burn dietary fat
- Increases endurance and energy levels
- Increases strength
- Improves sensitivity to insulin
- Reduces risk of diabetes

Mental Processes
- Provides a natural release for pent-up feelings
- Helps reduce tension and anxiety
- Improves mental outlook and self-esteem
- Helps relieve moderate depression
- Improves the ability to handle stress
- Stimulates improved mental function
- Relaxes and improves sleep
- Increases self-esteem

Longevity
- Promotes longevity

Physical Fitness and Longevity

The better shape that you are in physically, the greater your odds of enjoying a healthier and longer life. Most studies have shown that the risk of having a heart attack or stroke in an unfit individual is eight times greater than in a physically fit individual. Researchers have estimated that for every hour of exercise, there is a two-hour increase in longevity. That is quite a return on an investment.

Studies on physical fitness and mortality rate have historically relied on a single initial assessment of fitness, with subsequent follow-up for mortality. Unfortunately with such single-exposure assessments, there is no determinant of change in fitness or activity level. To counteract this deficiency in the medical research, there are several long-term studies in progress. Recent results from two of these studies, the Aerobics Center Longitudinal Study and the Harvard Alumni Health Study, provide further documentation on the benefits of being physically fit in reducing cardiovascular as well as all-cause mortality.

The Aerobics Center Longitudinal Study participants comprised 9,777 men ranging in age from twenty to eighty-two who had completed at least two preventive medical examinations at the Cooper Clinic in Dallas, Texas, from

December 1970 through December 1989. All study subjects achieved at least 85 percent of their age-predicted maximal heart rate (220 minus their age) during the treadmill tests at both exams. The average interval between the two exams was 4.9 years. Men were considered healthy if, in addition to normal resting and exercise electrocardiogram (EKG), they had no history or evidence of heart attack, stroke, diabetes, or high blood pressure at both exams. Men were considered unhealthy if they had one or more or these conditions, even though they had normal resting and exercising EKGs. A total of 6,819 men were classified as healthy and 2,958 unhealthy.[6]

Even though by standard definition all men in the study could be classified as being fit, for the purpose of category analysis, the men were further categorized by their level of fitness based on their exercise tolerance to a standard treadmill test. This measure is a sound objective indicator of physical fitness, as test time has been shown to correlate positively with maximal oxygen uptake. The men were divided into five groups, with the first quintile being labeled as unfit and quintiles 2 through 5 being categorized as fit.

The highest age-adjusted death rate (all causes) was observed in men who were unfit at both exams (122.0 deaths per 10,000 man-years); the lowest death rate was in men who were physically fit at both examinations (39.6 deaths per 10,000 man-years). Furthermore men who improved from unfit to fit between the first and subsequent examinations had an age-adjusted death rate of 67.7 per 10,000 man-years, representing a reduction in mortality of 44 percent relative to men who remained unfit at both exams. Improvement in fitness was associated with lower death rates after adjusting for age, health status, and other risk factors for premature mortality. For each minute increase in maximal treadmill time between examinations, there was a corresponding 7.9 percent decrease in risk of mortality.

The Harvard Alumni Health Study also demonstrated a good inverse relationship between total physical activity and all-cause mortality. The higher the activity level, the lower the death rate.[7]

Seven Steps to a Successful Exercise Program

Exercise is clearly one of the most powerful medicines available. Just imagine if all of the benefits of exercise could be put into a pill. Unfortunately it is not that easy. The time you spend exercising is a valuable investment toward good health. To help you develop a successful exercise program, here are seven steps to follow, taken from *Seven Keys to Vibrant Health*, by Terry Lemerond (Impakt Communications, Green Bay, WI, 1995):

Step 1. Realize the importance of physical exercise.

The first step is realizing just how vital exercise is to your health.

Step 2. Consult your physician.

If you are not currently on a regular exercise program, get medical clearance if you have health problems or if you are over forty years of age. The main concern is the functioning of your heart. Exercise can be quite harmful (even fatal) if your heart is not able to meet the increased demands placed upon it.

It is especially important to see a physician if any of the following applies to you:

Heart disease

Smoking

High blood pressure

Extreme breathlessness with physical exertion

Pain or pressure in chest, arm, teeth, jaw, or neck with exercise

Dizziness or fainting

Abnormal heart action (palpitations or irregular heartbeat)

Step 3. Select an activity you can enjoy.

If you are fit enough to begin, the next thing to do is to select an activity that you feel you would enjoy. Most authorities tell us that the best exercises are the kind that get your heart rate in the training range of 60 to 70 percent of your maximum heart rate. A quick and easy way to determine your maximum training heart rate is to simply subtract your age from 185. For example, if you are forty years old your maximum heart rate would be 145. To determine the bottom of the training zone, simply subtract 20 from this number. In the case of a forty-year-old this would be 125. So the training range would be a heart beat between 125 and 145 beats per minute. For maximum health benefits you must stay in this range and never exceed it. Aerobic activities such as walking briskly, jogging, bicycling, cross-country skiing, swimming, aerobic dance, and racquet sports are good examples. However, weight training is also of great benefit because it works to increase the amount of muscle tissue—the body's fat-burning machine. So weight training is also an option.[8]

For most people, brisk walking (five miles an hour) for approximately thirty minutes may be the very best form of exercise. Walking can be done anywhere; it doesn't require any expensive equipment, just comfortable clothing and well-fitting shoes; and the risk for injury is extremely low. If you are going to walk on a regular basis, I urge you to first purchase a pair of high-quality walking or jogging shoes. You'll be more comfortable, so you'll enjoy yourself more and will soon find you're walking longer and more frequently.

Consider joining a health club. I recommend it. You'll probably find it easier to stay motivated because you'll see other people working out hard. Don't be jealous of these people who are in phenomenal shape. Use them as motivation and as role models. A good health club will offer services and programs that can help you. Here are five tips to help you get the most out of your membership:

1. Take advantage of any personalized instruction that is available. A good health club should offer personalized supervision of at least your first few workouts in order to familiarize you with the different weight-lifting machines.

2. Get a personal trainer or workout partner for weight lifting. At most health clubs having a personal trainer supervise your workout costs extra. If you can afford it, it is well worth it. If you can't afford this luxury, find a good workout partner. A personal trainer or workout partner will increase your chance of success because he or she will push you.

3. Try different types of aerobics classes—low-impact, high-impact, Jazzercise, step, slide, cardio-funk, and so forth. Find several that you like, and vary your routine.

4. Try all of the different types of aerobic conditioning equipment—treadmills, bikes, stair machines, rowing machines, and so on—and find the one that you can enjoy doing.

5. Vary your routine. Don't get into the habit of doing the same thing every time you go to the club.

Step 4. Monitor exercise intensity.

Exercise intensity is determined by measuring your heart rate (the number of times your heart beats per minute). This can be quickly determined by placing the index and middle finger of one hand on the side of your neck just below the angle of the jaw or on the opposite wrist. Beginning with zero, count the number of heartbeats for six seconds. Simply add a zero to this number and you have your pulse. For example, if you counted fourteen beats, your heart rate would be 140. Would this be a good number? It depends upon your "training zone."

Step 5. Do it often.

You don't get in good physical condition by exercising once. Exercise must be performed on a regular basis. A minimum of fifteen to twenty minutes of exercising at your training heart rate at least three times a week is necessary to gain any significant cardiovascular benefits. For weight loss you will want to work out at least five days a week. Exercising at the lower end of your training zone for longer periods of time is much better than exercising at a higher intensity for a shorter period of time.

Step 6. Exercise with a friend.

Get a workout partner. For example, if you choose walking as your activity, find one or two people at work or in your neighborhood with whom you would enjoy walking. If you are meeting someone else, you will certainly walk more regularly than if no one is depending on you. Commit to walking three to five mornings or afternoons each week, and increase the exercise duration from an initial ten minutes to at least thirty minutes.

Step 7. Stay motivated.

No matter how committed a person is to regular exercise, at some point in time he or she is going to be faced with a loss of enthusiasm for working out. Here is my suggestion—take a break. Not a long break, just skip one or two workouts. Give your enthusiasm and motivation a chance to recoup so that you can come back with an even stronger commitment.

Here are some suggestions to help you stay motivated:

• Read or thumb through fitness magazines. Looking at pictures of people in fantastic shape is really inspirational. In addition these magazines typically feature articles on interesting new exercise routines.

• Set exercise goals. Goals really help with continued motivation. Write down your daily exercise goal and check it off when you have completed it.

• Vary your routine. Variety is very important to keep exercise interesting. Doing the same thing every day becomes monotonous and drains motivation. Continually find new ways to enjoy working out.

• Keep a record of your activities and progress. Sometimes it is hard to see the progress you are making, but if you write in a journal, you'll have a permanent record of your progress. Seeing your progress in black and white will motivate you to continued improvement.

Final Comments

Exercise is a critical component of a successful w
program as well as of good health. The benefits of ex
are tremendous, especially for the cardiovascular system. Th
key to achieving the benefits of exercise is to do it often at
the proper training intensity. For the long term it is important
to make exercise fun, vary the program, and stay motivated.

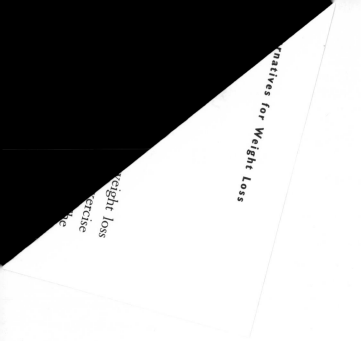

As stated many times in this book, one of the key goals for enhancing weight loss is to increase the sensitivity of cells throughout the body to the hormone insulin. Insulin plays a critical role in maintaining proper blood sugar levels as well as stimulating thermogenesis.

Here is how the body controls proper blood sugar levels: After a meal the body responds to the rise in blood glucose levels by secreting insulin. Insulin lowers blood glucose by increasing the rate that glucose is taken up by cells throughout the body. Declines in blood glucose, as occur during food deprivation or exercise, cause the release of glucagon—another hormone produced by the pancreas. Glucagon stimulates the release of glucose stored in body tissues as glycogen, especially the liver. If blood sugar levels fall sharply or if a person is angry or frightened, it may result in the release of epinephrine (adrenaline) and corticosteroids (cortisol) by the adrenal glands. These hormones provide quicker breakdown of stored glucose for extra energy during a crisis or increased need.

Ideally this is how the body works to control blood sugar levels. Unfortunately a great deal of Americans stress these control mechanisms through poor diet and lifestyle. As a result diabetes and hypoglycemia are among the most common of our diseases. Obesity is strongly linked to blood sugar disturbances as a result of decreased sensitivity to insulin. Increasing the body's sensitivity to insulin is associated not only with improved blood sugar control but also weight loss. The trace mineral chromium is essential in this goal.

Start with a High-Quality Multiple Vitamin and Mineral Formula

Chromium is not the only nutrient involved in proper insulin sensitivity and blood sugar control. A high-quality multiple vitamin and mineral formula will provide adequate levels of many of the key nutrients important for proper metabolism.

When you're shopping for a multiple, make sure it provides a full range of vitamins and minerals. Here are the optimum ranges to expect from a good multiple vitamin and mineral formula.

Vitamins:	Range for Adults
Vitamin A (retinol)	5,000 IU
Vitamin A (from beta-carotene)	5,000–25,000 IU
Vitamin D	100–400 IU
Vitamin E (d-alpha tocopherol)	400–800 IU
Vitamin K (phytonadione)	60–300 mcg
Vitamin C (ascorbic acid)	100–250 mg
Vitamin B_1 (thiamine)	10–100 mg
Vitamin B_2 (riboflavin)	10–100 mg
Niacin	10–100 mg
Niacinamide	10–30 mg
Vitamin B_6 (pyridoxine)	25–100 mg
Biotin	100–300 mcg
Pantothenic acid	25–100 mg
Folic acid	200–400 mcg
Vitamin B_{12}	200–400 mcg
Choline	10–100 mg
Inositol	10–100 mg

Minerals:	
Boron	1–2 mg
Calcium	250–750 mg
Chromium	200–400 mcg
Copper	1–2 mg

Iodine	50–150 mcg
Iron	15–30 mg
Magnesium	250–500 mg
Manganese	10–15 mg
Molybdenum	10–25 mcg
Potassium	200–500 mg
Selenium	100–200 mcg
Silica	200–1,000 mcg
Vanadium	50–100 mcg
Zinc	15–30 mg

In my clinical practice I use a formula that I developed for Enzymatic Therapy called Doctor's Choice. Because men and women have slightly different nutritional needs, I developed two versions: Doctor's Choice for Men and Doctor's Choice for Women. If you would like more information on these formulas or for a health food store near you that carries them, call Enzymatic Therapy at 1-800-783-2286.

Increasing Insulin Sensitivity with Chromium

The trace mineral chromium has gained a great deal of attention lately as a weight loss aid. The importance of this trace mineral in human nutrition was not discovered until 1957, when it was shown that it was essential to proper blood sugar control. Although there is no Recommended Dietary Allowance (RDA) for chromium, it appears that we need at least

200 mcg each day in our diet. Chromium levels can be depleted by refined sugars, white flour products, and lack of exercise.[1]

Chromium functions in the body as a key constituent of the "glucose tolerance factor." Chromium works closely with insulin in facilitating the uptake of glucose into cells. Without chromium, insulin's action is blocked and blood sugar levels are elevated.[1]

In some clinical studies in diabetics, supplementing the diet with chromium has been shown to decrease fasting glucose levels, improve glucose tolerance, lower insulin levels, and decrease total cholesterol and triglyceride levels, while increasing HDL-cholesterol levels.[2] Obviously chromium is a critical nutrient in diabetes, but it is also very important in hypoglycemia. In one study eight female patients with hypoglycemia given 200 micrograms a day for three months demonstrated alleviation of their symptoms of hypoglycemia.[3] In addition glucose tolerance test results were improved and the number of insulin receptors on red blood cells were increased.

Chromium supplementation has been demonstrated to lower body weight yet increase lean body mass, presumably as a result of increased insulin sensitivity.[4] In one study patients were given chromium bound to picolinic acid (chromium picolinate) in one of the following three doses daily for two and one-half months: 0 mcg (placebo), 200 mcg, or 400 mcg.[5] Patients taking the 200 mcg and 400 mcg dose lost an average of 4.2 pounds of fat. The group taking the placebo lost only 0.4 pounds. Even more impressive was the fact that the chromium groups gained more muscle (1.4 vs. 0.2 pounds) than those taking the placebo. The results were most striking in elderly subjects and in men. The men taking chromium picolinate lost more than seven times the amount of body fat than those taking the placebo (7.7 vs. 1 pound). The 400 mcg dose is more effective than the 200 mcg dose.

Effects of 200 mcg vs. 400 mcg per day
for 2½ months

Dosage	Fat Loss	Muscle gain	Total weight loss
200 mcg chromium picolinate	−3.3 lbs	+1.5 lbs	−1.8 lbs
400 mcg chromium picolinate	−4.6 lbs	+1.1 lbs	−3.5 lbs

The results of these preliminary studies with chromium are very encouraging. Particularly interesting is the fact that in these initial studies, chromium picolinate promoted an increase in lean body weight percentage as it led to fat loss, but increased the amount of lean body tissue, i.e., muscle.[6] Greater muscle mass means greater fat-burning potential.

All of the effects of chromium appear to be due to increased insulin sensitivity. There is evidence that marginal chromium deficiency is quite common in the United States. Chromium supplementation will often not only improve blood sugar control, but also lower cholesterol and triglyceride levels.[7]

Which Form of Chromium Is the Best?

There are several forms of chromium available on the market. Chromium picolinate, chromium polynicotinate, chromium chloride, and chromium-enriched yeast are each touted by their respective suppliers to provide the greatest benefit. Which is the best form? There really is no firm evidence to indicate that one is a significantly better choice than another, although there was one small study of six women and six men given either 400 micrograms of chromium picolinate or chromium polynicotinate. The test subjects were enrolled in an aerobics class for three months. Those taking the chromium picolinate increased muscle mass three times as much as those taking chromium polynicotinate (women: 4 lbs. vs. 1.3 lbs.; men: 4.6 lbs. vs. 1.5 lbs.).[6]

The current dosage recommendation for chromium as a weight loss aid that is being made by many experts in the field of nutritional medicine is 400 to 600 micrograms per day. Many manufacturers are now combining chromium with $(-)$-hydroxycitrate (discussed in Chapter 7).

Final Comments

Improving insulin sensitivity is an important goal in a weight loss program. Loss of insulin sensitivity is a hallmark feature of obesity. Chromium is a trace mineral necessary for the proper action of insulin on blood sugar control. Preliminary studies indicate that supplementing the diet with chromium can promote fat loss and muscle gain.

Chapter 6

Thermogenic Formulas

Herbal formulas and other compounds designed to promote diet-induced thermogenesis are among the most popular and controversial products in the nutritional supplement industry. When properly combined, these formulas can activate the sympathetic nervous system, thereby increasing the metabolic rate and thermogenesis. This effect results in weight loss by addressing the underlying defect in metabolism. The controversy surrounding these formulas centers around the side effects of ephedrine and caffeine, the major active components in these formulations. Ephedrine and caffeine combinations are not for everyone. However, they do appear to be quite useful in weight loss programs.

They absolutely must be used in a rational manner and not abused.

The Pharmacology of Ephedrine

Ephedrine, the major pharmacological alkaloid of *Ephedra sinica,* or ma huang, has a basic pharmacological action similar to that of adrenaline (epinephrine), although ephedrine is much less active. While adrenaline is not active when given orally, ephedrine is active orally. Ephedrine also has a longer duration of action and a more pronounced effect on the brain compared with adrenaline. The stimulatory effect on the brain caused by ephedrine is similar to those of amphetamines, but again much less potent.[1]

The cardiovascular effects of ephedrine are also similar to those of adrenaline, that is, ephedrine increases blood pressure, cardiac output, and heart rate but is much longer in duration (about ten times). Like adrenaline, ephedrine will also increase heart, brain, and muscle blood flow at the expense of kidney and intestinal blood flow.[2] Bronchial muscle as well as muscles of the uterus are also relaxed by ephedrine.[1]

Ephedrine in Weight Loss

Although ephedrine has demonstrated an appetite-suppressing effect, its main mechanism for promoting weight loss appears to be increasing the metabolic rate of fat tissue.[2] Its weight-reducing effects are greatest in those individuals with a low basal metabolic rate and/or decreased diet-induced thermogenesis.[3]

The thermogenic effects of ephedrine can be enhanced by methylxanthine compounds, such as caffeine and theophylline. Herbs rich in these active ingredients can be used in a fashion similar to isolated methylxanthines. Good methylxanthine sources include coffee *(Coffea arabica)*, tea *(Camellia sinensis)*, cola nut *(Cola nitida)*, and guarana *(Paullinea cupana)*. The optimum dosage of the crude plant preparation or extract depends on the content of active ingredient. Preparations standardized for caffeine content will produce more dependable results.

One study performed on animals sought to determine the weight-loss-promoting effects of ephedrine compared with a mixture of ephedrine and caffeine and/or theophylline. When ephedrine was used alone, it resulted in losses of 14 percent in body weight and 42 percent in body fat. However, when ephedrine was used in combination with caffeine or theophylline, there was a loss of 25 percent in body weight and 75 percent in body fat.[4] In contrast, when either caffeine or theophylline were used alone, there was no significant loss in body weight. The reason for the decrease in body weight is an increased metabolic rate and fat-cell breakdown promoted by ephedrine and enhanced by caffeine and theophylline.

Let's review some of the studies on weight loss using ephedrine alone and in combination with methylxanthines.

EPHEDRINE ONLY

Ephedrine as the sole agent in promoting weight loss has been the subject of several clinical studies.[5,6] The results have been inconsistent. For example, in one study overweight individuals were given either a placebo (group I), 25 mg of ephedrine (group II), or 50 mg of ephedrine (group III) three times daily for three months.[5] Dietary treatment consisted of 1,000 calories per day for females and 1,200 calories per day for males. Weight loss was similar in all groups. Patients in group III (ephedrine 150 mg/day) showed significantly more side effects than the placebo group.

In another study ten obese women were treated with a diet composed of 1,000 to 1,400 calories per day and either ephedrine (50 mg three times per day) or placebo for two months, and then switched treatments.[6] Weight loss was significantly greater during the ephedrine period (5.3 pounds) than during the placebo period (1.4 pounds).

The reason for these differences appears to be that ephedrine is effective primarily in those people with defects in diet-induced thermogenesis and ineffective in those without this defect. Overall the results seem to indicate that ephedrine as a sole agent is not as effective in promoting weight loss compared with products containing ephedrine combined with caffeine and/or theophylline even when ephedrine is given at a high daily dosage (e.g., 150 mg per day).

EPHEDRINE WITH METHYLXANTHINES

As mentioned above, the effectiveness of ephedrine in weight loss is greatly enhanced when it is combined with caffeine and/or theophylline. Most of the recent studies have used a combination providing 20 mg ephedrine and 200 mg of caffeine three times daily. Despite this very high dosage, long-term studies have shown good safety and efficacy.[7]

In one of the largest studies 180 overweight patients were treated by diet and either an ephedrine-caffeine combination (20mg/200mg), ephedrine (20 mg), caffeine (200 mg), or placebo three times a day for twenty-four weeks.[8] Average weight losses were greatest in the group given the ephedrine-caffeine combination. The ephedrine/caffeine group lost a [a total] of thirty six pounds as a group in twenty-four weeks compared with twenty-nine pounds for the placebo group. In the groups receiving ephedrine or caffeine only, weight loss was similar to that of the placebo group. Side effects (tremor, insomnia, and dizziness) were transient, and after eight weeks of treatment there was no difference in side effects in the group receiving the ephedrine-caffeine combination compared with the placebo group. Both systolic and diastolic blood pressure fell similarly in all four groups, indicating that the weight loss promoted by ephedrine and caffeine counteracted any increase in blood pressure these substances may promote.

Although more recent studies have used a daily dosage of 60 mg of ephedrine and 600 mg of caffeine, these high dosages may not be necessary. In one study a daily dosage of 22 mg ephedrine, 30 mg caffeine, and 50 mg theophylline was shown to greatly increase the basal metabolic rate and diet-induced thermogenesis.[9]

Fat Loss Versus Weight Loss

One of the key benefits of ephedrine-methylxanthine thermogenic formulas appears to be their ability to promote fat breakdown and not loss of lean muscle mass. For example one study of sixteen obese women on a weight-reducing diet given either a combination of ephedrine (20 mg) and caffeine (200 mg) twice daily or a placebo demonstrated no real significant differences in overall weight loss.[10] Both groups noted similar losses in total body weight. However, upon closer examination is was determined that the ephedrine-caffeine group lost 9.9 pounds more body fat and 6.16 pounds less lean body mass compared with the placebo group. These results indicate that ephedrine and caffeine combinations promote fat loss and preserve lean body mass during weight reduction diets. As an added bonus subjects in the study taking the ephedrine-caffeine combination had higher energy levels and burned more calories than the placebo group.

Comparison to D-fenfluramine

Drug companies have been investing hundreds of millions of dollars in the attempt to design the "perfect" diet pill. Some researchers have stated that D-fenfluramine is the closest thing available to the "magic bullet" for obesity. However, these researchers have not examined closely enough the studies that have shown that ephedrine-methylxanthine mixtures and several fiber supplements are often more effective and better tolerated.

D-fenfluramine is a prescription drug that is not yet FDA approved in the United States, although it has been used in Europe for many years. The drug works by reducing appetite. It is particularly effective in reducing the intake of high-carbohydrate foods. D-fenfluramine accomplishes this effect by increasing the level of serotonin in the brain, similar to the drug Prozac. D-fenfluramine has other effects that promote weight loss including enhancing diet-induced thermogenesis and energy expenditure during exercise. D-fenfluramine is not without side effects. Approximately 30 percent of all patients will experience one or more of the common side effects: fatigue (28%), diarrhea (15%), dry mouth (12%), increased urinary frequency (7%), and drowsiness (5%).[11]

In one study an ephedrine and caffeine combination was shown to be 20 to 29 percent more effective in promoting weight loss than D-fenfluramine.[12] A group of 103 patients who were 20 to 80 percent over their ideal body weight were put on a diet of 1,200 calories per day and given either the ephedrine-caffeine combination (20 mg and 200 mg, respectively) three times per day or 15 mg of D-fenfluramine twice daily for three and a half months. The group receiving the ephedrine-caffeine mixture lost an average 18.3 pounds while the group taking D-fenfluramine lost an average 15.2 pounds—a difference of 20 percent in favor of the ephedrine-caffeine combination. Furthermore, in a subgroup of patients who were greater than 40 percent above their ideal weight, the difference in weight loss in favor of the ephedrine-caffeine combination was 29 percent.

Ephedrine-Methylxanthine Combinations Versus OTC Weight Loss Aids

Ephedrine-methylxanthine mixtures have also shown to produce better results than over-the-counter (OTC) weight loss aids containing phenylpropanolamine (PPA). PPA is an amphetaminelike substance with milder stimulant effects that is the active ingredient in products such as Acutrim and Dexatrim. PPA is thought to promote weight loss by reducing the appetite, but this effect is debatable. The American Medical Association's Drug Evaluations states that PPA-containing products are only "minimally effective," and many standard pharmacology texts state that PPA is ineffective as an appetite suppressant.

How PPA was ever approved as a weight loss aid has been the subject of much interest. The FDA Advisory Review Panel admitted that the studies they used to base their decision were flawed—and they were also unpublished. The panel's approval of PPA has been severely criticized by many medical experts, who feel that the use of PPA poses a danger to the public. While the panel recommended a daily dosage of 150 milligrams, the maximum dosage that the FDA would sanction was 75 milligrams.

Side effects with PPA are common, especially if the recommended dosage is exceeded. Nervousness, restlessness, insomnia, headache, nausea, and elevations of blood pressure are some of PPA's adverse effects. People taking PPA should monitor their blood pressure, as PPA can produce severe elevations, even in people with normal blood pressure. People with high blood pressure, diabetes, thyroid disease, and depression should not take PPA unless under the supervision of a physician.

Another approved OTC weight loss aid that is not nearly as effective as ephedrine-methylxanthine mixtures is benzocaine. Benzocaine is an anesthetic that is incorporated into chewing gum, lozenge, or candy as a weight loss aid. Benzocaine is supposed to act to reduce appetite by numbing the taste receptors on the tongue. Since one of the reasons we eat is because we like the taste of food, the belief is that chewing gum or eating candy containing benzocaine will lead to less food being consumed. Although this sounds reasonable, benzocaine as an appetite suppressant has even less scientific support than PPA.

A Close Look at the Side Effects

Thermogenic formulas containing ephedrine and caffeine combinations can produce increased blood pressure, increased heart rate, insomnia, and anxiety. The FDA Advisory Review Panel on Nonprescription Drugs recommends that ephedrine not be taken by people with heart disease, high blood pressure, thyroid disease, diabetes, or difficulty in urination due to enlargement of the prostate. In addition ephedrine should not be used in people on blood-pressure-lowering drugs or antidepressants.

There is tremendous variation in the response to ephedrine and caffeine. Some people can tolerate high levels quite easily, whereas others are extremely sensitive to the stimulatory effects and will likely experience nervousness and/or insomnia.

It is interesting to examine the side effects reported in the studies using a daily dosage of 60 milligrams of ephedrine and 600 milligrams of caffeine. Surprisingly side effects were relatively mild. Although at week four 60 percent of subjects taking the ephedrine-caffeine combination typically reported side effects such as dizziness, headache, insomnia, heart palpitations, and headache, by week 8 the rate of side effects was substantially reduced. In fact just as many people in the placebo group reported symptoms compared with the group receiving ephedrine and caffeine.

There were other interesting findings in these studies. As stated above, systolic and diastolic blood pressure decreased, indicating that the effect of weight loss more than compensated any increase in blood pressure caused by the ephedrine and caffeine. Blood glucose, triglycerides, and cholesterol levels also decreased with weight loss and were not affected by ephedrine and caffeine.

Subjects taking the high doses of ephedrine and caffeine experienced withdrawal symptoms (hunger, tiredness, and headache) slightly more often than subjects taking placebo.

What About "Adrenal Exhaustion"?

It is believed by many people that if ephedrine is used over a long period, it may lose its effectiveness due to weakening of the adrenal glands. But according to the American Pharmaceutical Association, "There is far more discussion of ephedrine tachyphylaxis (rapid decrease in effectiveness) or tolerance than is evidenced as a significant problem in the scientific literature."[13] A 1977 study of ephedrine therapy in asthmatic children published in JAMA concluded, "Ephedrine is a potent bronchodilator that, in appropriate doses, can be administered safely along with therapeutic doses of theophylline without the fear of progressive tolerance or toxicity."[14]

Nonetheless many practitioners of natural medicine will often use ephedra in combination with substances that will support the adrenal glands, such as licorice *(Glycyrrhiza glabra)* and Panax ginseng and/or supplemental levels of vitamin C, magnesium, zinc, vitamin B6, and pantothenic acid.

What About Aspirin?

Some companies marketing thermogenic formulas add willow bark extracts or aspirin to their formulas in order to enhance the effect of the ephedrine/methylxanthine combination. I question this practice for several reasons. Before a physician prescribes any agent, or before anyone takes a medication, vitamin, mineral herb, or any other substance, an important question has to be asked: Does the benefit outweigh the risks? Do the benefits of aspirin outweigh the risks? First of all, what are the benefits? Clinical studies where subjects took 300 mg of aspirin along with ephedrine (75–150 mg) and caffeine (150 mg) have not demonstrated any greater benefit compared with ephedrine-caffeine combinations.[15] So, to answer the first part of our question, aspirin does not seem to offer any significant advantage compared with ephedrine-methylxanthine alone. Since the dosage of aspirin required (greater than 300 mg) is fairly high, it is simply not feasible to utilize willow bark for this purpose. Its inclusion in thermogenic formulas is purely for marketing purposes.

Given that aspirin does not offer any significant benefit;

what about the risk? Many side effects of aspirin are well known—gastric irritation, ulcer formation, and blood loss, for example. But there are other side effects. Aspirin is not as benign a drug as it was once thought.

Recently a detailed study evaluated the risk of gastrointestinal bleeding due to peptic ulcers caused by aspirin at daily dosages of 300 mg, 150 mg, and 75 mg. The study, conducted at five test hospitals in England, concluded an increased risk of gastrointestinal bleeding due to peptic ulcer at all dosage levels. However, the dosage of 75 mg per day was associated with a 40 percent reduction compared with 300 mg per day, and 30 percent for 150 mg per day. The researchers concluded, "No conventionally used prophylactic aspirin regimen seems free of the risk of peptic ulcer complications."[16]

It should be quite obvious that aspirin and willow bark extracts do not increase the effectiveness of ephedrine and methylxanthine preparations, yet they do possess significant risk of side effects. I see no reason to take aspirin in a thermogenic formula.

Final Comments

Permanent weight loss requires permanent changes in diet and lifestyle. Relying on thermogenic formulas alone to achieve weight loss goals is a quick fix at best and certainly not a part of lasting weight loss. Thermogenic formulas should be viewed as "crutches" until weight loss goals are achieved through a combination of diet and exercise. Thermogenic formulas can be quite useful in weight management because they address the underlying defect of impaired diet-induced thermogenesis.

In order to produce the desired weight loss benefit, herbal products containing ephedrine and caffeine must be used at the right dosage. Products standardized for their stimulant levels offer considerable benefits over herbal products, which do not specify the level of ephedrine or caffeine. Although recent studies have utilized high daily dosages of ephedrine (60 mg) and caffeine (600 mg), lower dosages (e.g., 30 mg ephedrine and 100 mg caffeine) may provide similar weight loss benefits and fewer side effects.

Chapter 7

Other Natural Weight Loss Promoters

There are several other natural weight loss aids that can be very useful in helping either reduce appetite or enhance metabolism. In order of effect, I would rate these items as follows:

Fiber supplements
Lipotropic compounds
Pancreatin
Medium-chain triglycerides
Hydroxycitrate
Carnitine, pantethine, and coenzyme Q10

Thyroid hormone

Meal replacement formulas

The effect and safe use of each of these natural weight loss aids will be described.

Fiber Supplements

The best fiber sources to use for weight loss are psyllium, guar gum, glucomannan, gum karaya, and pectin because they are rich in water-soluble fibers. When taken with water before meals, these fiber sources bind to the water in the stomach to form a gelatinous mass that makes you feel full. As a result you will be less likely to overeat.

The benefits of fiber go well beyond this mechanical effect, however. Fiber supplements have been shown to enhance blood sugar control and insulin effects, as well as actually reduce the number of calories absorbed by the body.[1] In some of the clinical studies demonstrating weight loss, fiber supplements were shown to reduce the number of calories absorbed by 30 to 180 calories per day.[2] This reduction in calories may not seem like much, but over the course of a year it would add up to three to eighteen pounds.

In addition to weight loss, fiber supplementation promotes good health. Studies have shown these very same water-soluble fiber sources to reduce the risk of heart disease by lowering cholesterol levels and lowering blood pressure; reduce the risk for various cancers including colon, rectal, and pancreatic cancer; reduce blood sugar levels in diabetes; promote proper bowel function; and help heal peptic ulcers.

There are many fiber supplements to choose from in health food stores. The only recommendation I will make is to select a product that is rich in water-soluble fiber and avoid products that add a lot of sugar or other sweeteners to camouflage the taste. One other very important recommendation is to be sure to drink adequate amounts of water when taking any fiber supplement, especially if it is in a pill form. If you have a disorder of the esophagus, do not take fiber supplements in a pill form, as they may expand in the esophagus and lead to obstruction of the intestinal tract, a very serious disorder.[3] Fiber supplements in capsules appear to be slightly better tolerated than tablets, but still should be used with caution. The difference is in how the tablets and capsules interact with water. One study showed that fiber (glucomannan) tablets swelled seven times their original size within one minute after coming in contact with water.[4] By contrast, fiber-filled gelatin capsules took six minutes before they began to swell.

How much fiber should you take and how much weight can you expect to lose by taking a fiber supplement? Let's take a look at the weight loss studies with fiber supplements.

The most impressive results in weight loss studies have been achieved with guar gum, a water-soluble fiber obtained from the Indian cluster bean *(Cyamopsis tetragonoloba)*. In one study nine women weighing between 160 and 242 pounds were given 10 grams of guar gum immediately before lunch

Clinical Studies with Dietary Fiber Supplements[5-14]

Fiber	Number of subjects	Length of study	Dosage	Calorie restriction	Avg. loss w/fiber	Avg. loss w/placebo	Reference
Guar	9	2 months	20 g/day	None	9.4 lbs	No placebo group	5
Guar	7	1 year	20 g/day	None	61.9 lbs	No placebo group	6
Guar	21	2½ months	20 g/day	None	15.6 lbs	No placebo group	7
Guar	33	2.5 months	15 g/day	None	5.5 lbs	0.9 lbs in placebo group	8
Glucomannan	20	2 months	3 g/day	None	5.5 lbs	Weight gain of 1.5 lbs	9
Glucomannan	20	2 months	3 g/day	None	8.14 lbs	0.44 lbs in placebo group	10
Citrus Pectin	14	4 weeks	5.56 g/day	Yes	12.8 lbs	No placebo group	11
Mixture A	60	12 weeks	5 g/day	Yes	18.7 lbs	14.7 lbs in placebo group	12
Mixture A	89	11 weeks	10 g/day	Yes	13.9 lbs	9.2 lbs in placebo group	13
Mixture B	45	3 months	7 g/day	Yes	13.6 lbs	9 lbs in placebo group	14
Mixture B	97	3 months	7 g/day	Yes	10.8 lbs	7.3 lbs in placebo group	5
Mixture B	52	6 months	7 g/day	Yes	12.1 lbs	6.1 lbs in placebo group	1

Mixture A = 80% fiber from grains, 20% fiber from citrus; Mixture B = 90% insoluble and 10% soluble fiber from beet, barley, and citrus fibers.

and dinner. They were told not to consciously alter their eating habits. After two months the women reported an average weight loss of 9.4 pounds—over 1 pound per week. Reductions were also noted for cholesterol and triglyceride levels.[15]

Studies with soluble fiber in the treatment of elevated cholesterol levels have shown a dose-dependent effect—the higher the dosage, the greater the cholesterol-lowering effect.[16] Dietary fiber supplements appear to exert a dose-dependent effect in weight loss studies as well. Therefore to achieve the greatest benefit, the dosage should be as high as possible.

A word of caution: Start out with a small dosage and increase gradually. Water-soluble fibers are fermented by intestinal bacteria. As a result a great deal of gas can be produced. If you are not used to a high-fiber diet, an increase in dietary fiber can lead to increased flatulence and abdominal discomfort. Start out with a dosage between 1 and 2 grams before meals and at bedtime and gradually increase the dosage to 5 grams. How much weight will you lose? It really depends on how much you weigh, but based on all of the studies with fiber and weight loss, you should lose 50 to 100 percent more weight by supplementing your diet with fiber than by simply restricting calories alone.

Lipotropic Compounds

The liver's ability to break down and metabolize fat is impaired in a very large percentage of overweight individuals.[17] This liver dysfunction can be improved by using nutritional factors known as *lipotropic agents.* Lipotropic agents are compounds that promote the flow of fat and bile to and from the liver. In essence they produce a "decongesting" effect on the liver and promote improved liver function and fat metabolism. Examples of commonly used lipotropic compounds are choline, methionine, betaine, and inositol.

Formulas containing lipotropic agents are also very useful in enhancing detoxification reactions. As a result lipotropic formulas have been used by nutrition-oriented physicians for a wide variety of conditions including a number of liver disorders, such as hepatitis and cirrhosis.

I recommend using formulas that supply a number of lipotropic agents rather than just choline or methionine. When looking for a formula make sure that it can easily provide a daily dosage of 1,000 mg total of a combination of choline, betaine, inositol, and methionine. Such formulas are available in health food stores (e.g., Liv-A-Tox from Enzymatic Therapy, Lipotropic Complex from Nature's Life, and Lipotropic Factors from Solgar).

Pancreatin

Pancreatin is a powdered preparation of desiccated and de-fatted raw pancreas from pigs that is often used to supplement digestive enzyme deficiencies. Pancreatin supplementation has been shown to result in decreased food intake and a significant loss of body weight in animals.[18] Pancreatin appears to either contain or stimulate the manufacture of compounds that suppress appetite.

Although to my knowledge there are no human studies with pancreatin as a weight loss aid, I have seen pancreatin supplementation promote dramatic weight loss. The best example I can think of is a friend of mine, Jim, who lost at least forty pounds, and six inches around his waist, simply by supplementing his diet with pancreatin. Jim decided to try pancreatin because he was extremely sensitive to ephedrine and could not use thermogenic formulas.

For maximum benefit it is best to use a full-strength undiluted pancreatic extract (8–10X U.S.P.), as lower-potency pancreatin products are often diluted with salt, lactose, or galactose. Take 250 to 500 milligrams of full-strength pancreatin before meals or whenever you feel hungry.

For individuals wanting a vegetarian source of enzymes, bromelain (the enzyme complex from pineapple) can be used at a dosage of 500 to 750 milligrams before meals or whenever you feel hungry.

Medium-Chain Triglycerides

Medium-chain triglycerides (MCTs) are special types of saturated fats separated out from coconut oil that range in length from 6 to 12 carbon chains. MCTs are used by the body differently from the long-chain triglycerides (LCTs), which are the most abundant fats found in nature. LCTs are the storage fat for both humans and plants that range in length from 18 to 24 carbons. This difference in length makes all the difference in how MCTs and LCTs are utilized. Unlike regular fats, MCTs do not appear to cause weight gain, they actually promote weight loss.

MCTs accomplish this weight loss "magic" by increasing thermogenesis. In contrast, the LCTs are usually stored in the fat deposits, and since their energy is conserved, a high-fat diet actually decreases the metabolic rate. The reason for the difference in how the body handles MCTs versus LCTs is due to their size. The larger LCTs are difficult for the body to metabolize, so the body tends to want to store these fats. MCTs, on the other hand, are rapidly burned as energy and actually promote the burning of LCTs.[19]

A friend of mine, Dr. Julian Whitaker, has an interesting analogy: LCTs are like heavy, wet logs that you put on a small campfire. Keep adding the logs, and soon you have more logs than fire. MCTs are like rolled-up newspaper soaked in gasoline. Not only do they burn brightly but they will burn up the wet logs as well.

Scientific studies appear to support Dr. Whitaker's view. In one study the thermogenic effect of a high-calorie diet containing 40 percent fat as MCTs was compared with one containing 40 percent fat as LCTs.[20] The thermogenic effect (calories wasted six hours after meal) of the MCTs was almost twice as high as the LCTs, 120 calories versus 66 calories. The researchers concluded that the excess energy provided by fats in the form of medium-chain triglycerides would not be efficiently stored as fat but rather would be burned. A follow-up study demonstrated that MCT oil given over a six-day period can increase diet-induced thermogenesis by 50 percent.[21]

In another study, researchers compared single meals of 400 calories composed entirely of MCTs or LTCs.[22] The thermic effect of MCTs over six hours was three times greater than that of LCTs. In addition, while the LCTs elevated blood fat levels by 68 percent, MCTs had no effect on the blood fat level. Researchers concluded that substituting MCTs for LCTs would produce weight loss as long as the calorie level remained the same.

In order to gain the benefit from MCTs, a diet must remain low in LCTs. MCTs can be used as an oil for salad dressing, a bread spread, or simply taken as a supplement. A good dosage recommendation for MCTs is one to two tablespoons per day. MCTs are available in your health food store. Several companies mix in an orange flavor. Typically these products are available at health food stores and cost approximately $11.00 to $12.00 for a 16-ounce bottle.

Sound Nutrition, Inc., a company based in Dover, Idaho, has developed a patent-pending method of flavoring MCTs. Their product is Thin Oil and it is available as Original, Buttery Flavored, Olive Oil Flavored, and Garlic Flavored. Thin Oil can be used in salad dressings, as a bread spread, over pasta and popcorn, and in baked goods. Thin Oil is available in some health food stores as well as directly from the company by calling 1-800-844-6645.

WARNING: Diabetics and individuals with liver disease should not use MCTs unless under a doctor's supervision.

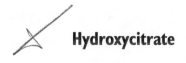 **Hydroxycitrate**

Hydroxycitrate is a natural substance isolated from the fruit of the Malabar tamarind *(Garcinia cambogia)*. It is a powerful lipogenic inhibitor (*lipo* means "fat," *-genic* means "production," so *lipogenic* means "fat production"). Therefore a lipogenic inhibitor is a substance that helps prevent the production of fat.

The Malabar tamarind is a yellowish fruit that is about the size of an orange, with a thin skin, and deep furrows similar to an acorn squash. It is native to southern India, where it is dried and used extensively in curries. The dried fruit contains about 30 percent hydroxycitric acid.

Hydroxycitrate has been shown to be a powerful inhibitor of fat formation in animals.[23] Whether or not it demonstrates this effect in humans is not yet proven. The weight-loss–promoting effects in animals are perhaps best exemplified in a study that shows hydroxycitrate producing a "significant reduction in food intake, and body weight gain" in rats.[24] Hydroxycitrate may not only be a powerful inhibitor of fat production, it may also suppress appetite.

It is critical when using a hydroxycitrate formula that a low-fat diet be maintained. Hydroxycitrate only inhibits the conversion of carbohydrates into fat. Therefore it will have no effect if a high-fat diet is consumed.

On its own hydroxycitrate may offer a safe, natural aid for weight loss when taken at a dosage of 500 milligrams three times daily. However by combining it with chromium and a thermogenic formula an even greater effect may be noted because in addition to inhibiting the production of fat, there is also an increase in the burning of fat.

Carnitine, Pantethine, and Coenzyme Q10

These three compounds are essential in the proper transport and breakdown of fat into energy. Clinical studies have shown that all three of these nutritional factors are useful in lowering blood cholesterol and triglyceride levels and are of extreme benefit to sufferers of angina and other heart disturbances. Studies have also shown they may help promote weight loss. For example in one study coenzyme Q10 levels were found to be low in 52 percent (fourteen out of twenty-seven) of overweight subjects tested.[25] Nine subjects (five with low CoQ10 levels, four with normal levels) were given 100 mg/day of CoQ10 along with a low-calorie diet. After nine weeks mean weight loss in the CoQ10-deficient group was 29.7 pounds compared with 12.76 in those with initially normal levels of CoQ10. This study suggests that about 50 percent of overweight individuals may be deficient in CoQ10, and that treatment with 100 mg/day of CoQ10 may accelerate weight loss resulting from a low-calorie diet.

The dosage for carnitine and pantethine as weight loss aids is 300 milligrams each three times daily. The drawback of these three compounds is that they are relatively expensive. Unless you can afford the $100 per month these supplements are likely to cost, my recommendation is to use them only if you are doing everything else and nothing seems to be helping. The reason nothing else may be working is an underlying deficiency of either carnitine, pantethine, or coenzyme Q10. Because they work together and it is difficult to determine which factor a person may be deficient in, I would recommend using all three at the suggested dosages for at least two months. If you are deficient in one of the three fat-burning nutrients, you should experience dramatic weight loss (at least twice the rate of your previous weight loss rate) by including them in your diet.

Thyroid Hormone

Significant obesity is one of the hallmark features of an under-active thyroid. Since the thyroid gland controls metabolism, it makes sense that low thyroid function (hypothyroidism) con-tributes to weight gain. One of the easiest and most accurate assessments of thyroid function is measurement of the temper-ature of the body while at rest—the basal body temperature. Body temperature reflects metabolic rate. This rate is largely determined by hormones secreted by the thyroid gland. Many physicians and experts in endocrinology believe that measuring the level of thyroid hormones in the blood does not accurately diagnose hypothyroidism. To measure basal body temperature, you will need a thermometer.

MEASURING YOUR BASAL BODY TEMPERATURE

1. Shake down the thermometer to below 95 degrees F and place it by your bed before going to sleep at night.

2. On waking, place the thermometer in your armpit for a full ten minutes. It is important to make as little move-ment as possible. Remaining lying down and resting with your eyes closed is best. Do not get up until the ten-minute test is completed.

3. After ten minutes read and record the temperature and date.

4. Record the temperature for at least three mornings (preferably at the same time of day) and give the information to your physician. Menstruating women must perform the test on the second, third, and fourth days of menstruation because of the natural temperature fluctuations due to the menstrual cycle. Men and postmenopausal women can perform the test at any time.

INTERPRETATION

Your basal body temperature should be between 97.6 and 98.2 degrees F. The reason it is below the "normal" of 98.6 degrees is that you are taking your temperature under the arm rather than orally or anally. Temperature registers roughly a point lower in this spot. Note that low basal body temperatures are quite common. They do not prove hypothyroidism. [It is more likely that a thyroid problem is behind your low temperature if you also have some of the symptoms associated with hypothyroidism, such as difficulty losing weight, dry skin, depression, and cold hands or feet.]

High basal body temperatures (above 98.6 degrees F) are less common. They may be evidence of hyperthyroidism. Common signs and symptoms of hyperthyroidism include bulging eyeballs, fast pulse, hyperactivity, inability to gain weight, insomnia, irritability, menstrual problems, and nervousness. In short the symptoms of hyperthyroidism tend to be what would reasonably be associated with heating up or speeding up the body.

THYROID HORMONES AND WEIGHT LOSS

The use of thyroid hormones in cases of hypothyroidism confirmed by low blood levels of thyroid hormones is well-accepted medical practice. However, the use of thyroid hormone therapy in individuals with low basal body temperatures is extremely controversial, as is prescribing thyroid hormone to stimulate metabolism and promote weight loss. My recommendation is if your basal body temperature is low and you want to lose weight, definitely find a physician willing to prescribe thyroid hormone. My reasoning is that there are several studies that have demonstrated that thyroid hormone supplementation can effectively accelerate weight loss and is extremely useful in overcoming the adaptive decreased metabolic rate associated with prolonged dieting.[26] Thyroid hormone medications must be prescribed by a physician. I recommend the natural thyroid preparations over the synthetic ones, such as Synthroid.

If your body temperature was between 97.2 and 97.8 degrees, you may be helped by thyroid preparations sold in health food stores. While the FDA prohibits any thyroxine in these products, it is actually virtually impossible for a manufacturer to entirely remove thyroxine. In a sense the health-food-store thyroid formulas are mild forms of desiccated natural thyroid. Manufacturers will usually enhance these formulas with additional thyroid support, such as iodine, zinc, and tyrosine. You can use the basal body temperature test to monitor effectiveness of these formulas.

Using Meal Replacement Formulas

Meal replacement formulas that mix with water, juice, or milk are popular weight loss aids. The drink mixture is used to replace a meal. While these formulas can provide short-term benefit, in the long run a successful program must incorporate healthier food choices. There are numerous meal replacement formulas on the market. Here are five guidelines for choosing a healthy version:

1. Look for a product that contains high-quality protein. The best protein sources are from whey, hydrolyzed lactalbumin, and soy. Avoid nonfat milk and casein-based formulas. Casein, a milk protein, is often difficult for people to digest, many people are allergic to it, and it has been shown to raise blood cholesterol levels. Casein is used not only in many meal replacement formulas, it is also used in glues, molded plastics, and paints.

2. The formula should contain at least 5 grams of a combination of soluble and insoluble dietary fibers.

3. Look for balanced high-quality nutrition with enhanced levels of nutrients critical to weight loss such as chromium.

4. The formula should have low total fat content, but supply some essential fatty acids.

5. The formula should not contain sweeteners, artificial fla-

vors, or other artificial food additives. Refined sugar leads to loss of blood sugar control, diabetes, and obesity. Sucrose (white table sugar) is often the first ingredient of many meal replacement formulas.

Final Comments

Several natural aids to augment weight loss have been described. Impressive results have been obtained with fiber supplements, particularly soluble fiber sources such as guar gum, oat bran, and pectin. Many overweight individuals suffer from impaired liver function. Lipotropic formulas can improve liver function and may prove useful as weight loss aids. Carnitine, pantethine, and coenzyme Q10 are involved in the conversion of fat into energy. Preliminary studies indicate these compounds can help with weight loss in certain individuals. Proper thyroid function is essential to weight loss. Meal replacement formulas can help in the short term, but should be replaced with healthful food choices in the long term.

Chapter 8

Putting It All Together

If you have made it this far, you should have a clear vision of what you need to do to achieve your weight loss goals. This chapter will summarize the steps that you will need to take as well as more clearly guide you in the proper use of natural weight loss aids.

Step 1: Make the commitment to good health.

If you are absolutely, one-hundred-percent totally committed to achieving your goal, there is nothing that can keep you from attaining it. Make the commitment to be healthy, and renew that commitment every day!

Step 2: Eat a low-fat, high-fiber diet.

Permanent weight loss requires a lifelong commitment to eating a health-promoting diet that is low in fat and high in fiber-rich foods.

Step 3: Exercise.

Regular exercise is critical to achieving weight loss and maintaining health.

Step 4: Supplement your diet with chromium and a high-potency multiple vitamin-mineral formula.

Chromium can help improve blood sugar control. A high-potency multiple vitamin-mineral formula provides a good nutritional foundation.

Step 5: Use a thermogenic formula.

When used properly, thermogenic formulas containing ephedrine and methylxanthine mixtures can produce dramatic weight loss safely and effectively.

Step 6: Before each meal take a fiber supplement.

Water-soluble fiber not only reduces food intake but also lowers cholesterol levels and helps reduce the risk for cancers of the gastrointestinal tract.

Step 7: Use other natural weight loss aids if needed.

If additional support is needed, there are several other natural weight loss aids that may help. Particularly useful are lipotropic factors, which can help improve a sluggish metabolism due to impaired liver function, or medium-chain triglycerides, which can help stoke the metabolic fire.

There you have it—a natural prescription for achieving and maintaining your ideal body weight. The most critical component of this prescription is your commitment. Don't wait until your health is beyond repair. Make the commitment to be healthy right now and take the necessary steps to help you achieve the highest level of health possible. You can do it!

References

Preface

1. Kuczmarski, R., et al. Increasing prevalence of overweight among U.S. adults. *JAMA* 272:205–11, 1994.
2. Kolata, G. Obese children: A growing problem. *Science* 232:20–21, 1986.
3. Centers for Disease Control and Prevention. Prevalence of overweight among adolescents—United States, 1988–91. *MMWR Morb. Mortal. Wkly. Rep.* 43(44): 818–21, 1994.

Chapter I: Why Diets Don't Work

1. Gillum, R. F. The association of body fat distribution with hypertension, hypertensive heart disease, coronary heart disease, diabetes and cardiovascular risk factors in men and women aged 18–79 years. *J. Chron. Dis.* 40:421–8, 1987.
2. Dietz, W. H., and Gortmaker, S. L. Do we fatten our children at the television set? *Pediatrics* 75:807–12, 1985.
3. Tucker, L. A., and Bagwell, M. Television viewing and obesity in adult females. *Am. J. Public Health* 81:908–11, 1991.

4. Foreyt, J. P., et al. Behavioral treatment of obesity: Results and limitations. *Behavioral Therapy* 13:153–61, 1982.

5. Kolata, G. Why do people get fat? *Science* 227: 1327–28, 1985.

6. Bennett, W., and Gurin, J. *The dieter's dilemma.* Basic Books, New York, 1982.

7. National Research Council. *Diet and health. Implications for reducing chronic disease risk.* National Academy Press, Washington, D.C., 1989.

8. Vasselli, J. R., Cleary, M. P., and Van Itallie, T. B. Obesity. In *Present Knowledge in Nutrition,* 5th ed. Nutrition Foundation, Washington, D.C., 1984, pp. 45–49.

9. Hjermann, I. The metabolic cardiovascular syndrome: Syndrome X, Reaven's syndrome, insulin resistance syndrome, atherthrombogenic syndrome. *J. Cardiovascular Pharm.* 20(suppl. 8)S5–S10, 1992.

10. Maseri, A. Syndrome X: Still an appropriate name. *J. Am. Coll. Cardiol.* 17:1471–72, 1991.

11. Laville, M., et al. Decreased glucose-induced thermogenesis at the onset of obesity. *Am. J. Clin. Nutr.* 57:851–56, 1993.

12. Ravussin, E., et al. Evidence that insulin resistance is responsible for the decreased thermic effect of glucose in human obesity. *J. Clin. Invest.* 76:1268–73, 1985.

13. Astrup, A., Christensen, N. J., and Breum, L. Reduced plasma noradrenaline concentrations in simple-obese and diabetic obese patients. *Clin. Sci.* 80:53–58, 1991.

14. Nelson, K. M., et al. Effect of weight reduction on resting energy expenditure, substrate utilization, and the thermic effect of food in moderately obese women. *Am. J. Clin. Nutr.* 55:924–33, 1992.

15. Schultz, L. O. Brown adipose tissue: Regulation of thermogenesis and implications for obesity. *J. Am. Diet. Assoc.* 87:761–64, 1987.

16. Sims, E. A., et al. Endocrine and metabolic effects of experimental obesity in man. *Rec. Prog. Hor. Res.* 29:457–96, 1973.

17. Leibel, R. L., and Hirsch, J. Diminished energy requirements in reduced obese patients. *Metabolism* 33:164–70, 1984.

18. Eck, L. H. Children at familial risk for obesity: An examination of

dietary intake, physical activity, and weight status. *Int. J. Obes.* 16:
71–78, 1992.

19. Kawate, R., et al. Diabetes mellitus and its vascular complications in
    Japanese migrants on the island of Hawaii. *Diabetes Care* 2:161–70,
    1979.

Chapter 2: Making the Commitment

1. National Institutes of Health. Health implications of obesity. *Annals
   Int. Med.* 103:1073–77, 1985.

2. Lee, I. M., et al. Body weight and mortality. *JAMA* 270:2823–88,
   1993.

3. Lew, E. A., and Garfinkel, L. Variations in mortality by weight
   among 750,000 men and women. *J. Chronic Dis.* 32:563–66, 1979.

4. Lean, M. E., et al. Obesity, weight loss, and prognosis in type 2
   diabetics. *Diabetic Med.* 7:228–33, 1990.

Chapter 3: Dietary Guidelines

1. Anderson, J. Nutrition management in diabetes mellitus. In *Modern
   Nutrition in Health and Disease*, ed. Goodhart, R., and Young,
   V. R. Lea and Febiger, Philadelphia, 1988, pp. 1201–29.

2. Abbott, W. G., et al. Short-term energy balance: Relationship with
   protein, carbohydrate, and fat balances. *Am. J. Physiology* 255:E332–
   37, 1988.

3. Blundell, J. E., et al. Dietary fat and the control of energy intake:
   Evaluating the effects of fat on meal size and postmeal satiety. *Am.
   J. Clin. Nutr.* 57:772S–778S, 1993.

4. Lawton, C. L., et al. Dietary fat and appetite control in obese subjects:
   Weak effects on satiation and satiety. *Int. J. Obesity.* 17:409–16,
   1993.

5. Blundell, J. E., et al. Dietary fat and the control of energy intake:

Evaluating the effects of fat on meal size and postmeal satiety. *Am. J. Clin. Nutr.* 57 (suppl. 5):772S–778S, 1993.

6. Simpson, H.C.R., et al. A high carbohydrate leguminous fiber diet improves all aspects of diabetic control. *Lancet* 1:1–5, 1981

7. Cheng, K. K., et al. Pickled vegetables in the aetiology of oesophageal cancer in Hong Kong Chinese. *Lancet* 339:1314–18, 1992.

8. National Research Council. *Diet and health. Implications for reducing chronic disease risk*. National Academy Press, Washington, D.C., 1989.

9. Willett, W. C., et al. Intake of trans fatty acids and risk of coronary heart disease among women. *Lancet* 341:581–85, 1993.

    Longnecker, M. P. Do trans fatty acids in margarine and other foods increase the risk of coronary heart disease? *Epidemiology* 4: 492–95, 1993.

    Booyens, J., and Van Der Merwe, C. F. Margarines and coronary artery disease. *Med. Hypothesis* 37:241–44, 1992.

    Mensink, R. P., and Katan, M. B. Effect of dietary trans fatty acids on high-density and low-density lipoprotein cholesterol levels in healthy subjects. *New Eng. J. Med.* 323:439–45, 1990.

10. Pelikanova, T., et al. Fatty acid composition of serum lipids and erythrocyte membranes in type 2 (non-insulin-dependent) diabetic men. *Metab. Clin. Exp.* 40:175–80, 1991.

11. Borkman, M., et al. The relationship between insulin sensitivity and the fatty acid composition of skeletal-muscle phospholipids. *New Eng. J. Med.* 328:238–44, 1993.

    Pelikanova, T., et al. Insulin secretion and insulin action are related to the serum phospholipid fatty acid pattern in healthy men. *Metab. Clin. Exp.* 38:188–92, 1989.

12. Feskens, E. J. M., Bowles, C. H., and Kromhout, D. Inverse association between fish intake and risk of glucose intolerance in normoglycemic elderly men and women. *Diabetes Care* 14:935–41, 1991.

13. Storlien, L. H., et al. Influence of dietary fat composition on the development of insulin resistance in rats: Relation to muscle tri-

glyceride and omega-3 fatty acids in muscle phospholipid. *Diabetes* 40:280–89, 1991.

14. Vessby, B., et al. The risk to develop NIDDM is related to the fatty acid composition of the serum cholesterol esters. *Diabetes* 43:1353–57, 1994.

15. Fraser, G. E., et al. A possible protective effect of nut consumption on risk of coronary heart disease. *Arch. Intern. Med.* 152:1416–24, 1992.

16. Sabate, J., et al. Effect of walnuts on serum lipid levels and blood pressure in normal men. *New Eng. J. Med.* 328:603–607, 1993.

17. Beynen, A. C., Van der Meer, R., and West, C. E. Mechanism of casein-induced hypercholesterolemia: Primary and secondary features. *Atherosclerosis* 60:291–93, 1986.

18. Carrol, K. K. Review of clinical studies on cholesterol-lowering response to soy protein. *Journal of the American Dietetic Association* 91: 820–27, 1991.

19. Stanto, J. L., and Keast, D. R. Serum cholesterol, fat intake, and breakfast consumption in the United States adult population. *J. Am. Coll. Nutr.* 8:567–72, 1989.

Chapter 4: The Importance of Exercise

1. Pollack, M. L., Wilmore, J. H., and Fox, S. M. *Exercise in health and disease.* W. B. Saunders, Philadelphia, 1984.

2. Dietz, W. H., and Gortmaker, S. L. Do we fatten our children at the television set? *Pediatrics* 75:807–12, 1985.

3. Farmer, M. E., et al. Physical activity and depressive symptomatology: The NHANES 1 epidemiologic follow-up study. *Am. J. Epidemiol.* 1328:1340–51, 1988.

4. Daniel Carr, et al. Physical conditioning facilitates the exercise-induced secretion of beta-endorphin and beta-lipoprotein in women. *New Eng. J. Med.* 305:560–65, 1981.

5. Lobstein, D., Mosbacher, B. J., and Ismail, A. H. Depression as a

powerful discriminator between physically active and sedentary middle-aged men. *J. Psychosom. Res.* 27:69–76, 1983.

6. Blair, S. N., et al. Changes in physical fitness and all-cause mortality. A prospective study of healthy and unhealthy men. *JAMA* 273: 1093–98, 1995.

7. Lee, I. M., Hsieh, C. C., and Paffenbarger, R. S. Exercise intensity and longevity in men. The Harvard alumni health study. *JAMA* 273:1179–84, 1995.

8. Ballor, D. L., et al. Resistance weight training during calorie restriction enhances lean body weight maintenance. *Am. J. Clin. Nutr.* 47:19–25, 1988.

Chapter 5: Chromium

1. Mertz, W. Chromium in human nutrition: A review. *J. Nutr.* 123: 626–33, 1993.

2. Anderson, R. A. Chromium, glucose tolerance, and diabetes. *Biological Trace Element Research* 32:19–24, 1992.

3. Anderson, R. A., et al. Effects of supplemental chromium on patients with symptoms of reactive hypoglycemia. *Metabolism* 36:351–55, 1987.

4. McCarthy, M. F.: Hypothesis: Sensitization of insulin-dependent hypothalamic glucoreceptors may account for the fat-reducing effects of chromium picolinate. *J. Optimal Nutr.* 21:36–53, 1993.

5. Evans, G. W., and Pouchnik, D. J. Composition and biological activity of chromium-pyridine carbosylate complexes. *J. Inorgranic Biochemistry* 49:177–87, 1993.

   Katts, G. R., Ficher, J. A., and Blum, K. The effects of chromium picolinate supplementation on body composition in different age groups. *Age* 14:138 (abstract 40), 1991.

6. Evans, G. W. Chromium picolinate is an efficacious and safe supplement. *Int. J. Sport Nutr.* 3:117–22, 1993.

7. Press, R. I., Geller, J., and Evans, G. W. The effect of chromium

picolinate on serum cholesterol and apolipoprotein fractions in human subjects. *Western J. Med.* 152:41–45, 1993.

Chapter 6: Thermogenic Formulas

1. Gilman, A. G., Goodman, A. S., and Gilman, A. *The pharmacologic basis of therapeutics.* Macmillan Publishing, New York, 1980.
2. Astrup, A., et al. Pharmacology of thermogenic drugs. *Am. J. Clin. Nutr.* 55(suppl. 1):246S–248S, 1992.
3. Astrup, A., et al. The effect of chronic ephedrine treatment on substrate utilization, the sympathoadrenal activity, and expenditure during glucose-induced thermogenesis in man. *Metabolism* 35:260–65, 1986.
4. Dulloo, A. G., and Miller, D. S. The thermogenic properties of ephedrine/methylxanthine mixtures: Animal studies. *Am. J. Clin. Nutr.* 43:388–94, 1986.
5. Pasquali, R. A controlled trial using ephedrine in the treatment of obesity. *Int. J. Obes.* 9:93–98, 1985.
6. Pasquali, R., and Casimirri, F. Clinical aspects of ephedrine in the treatment of obesity. *Int. J. Obes.* 17(suppl. 1):S65–68, 1993.
7. Toubro, S., et al. Safety and efficacy of long-term treatment with ephedrine, caffeine and an ephedrine/caffeine mixture. *Int. J. Obes.* 17(suppl. 1):S69–72, 1993.
8. Astrup, A., et al. The effect and safety of an ephedrine/caffeine compound compared to ephedrine, caffeine and placebo in obese subjects on an energy restricted diet. A double blind trial. *Int. J. Obes.* 16:269–77, 1992.
9. Dulloo, A. G., and Miller, D. S. The thermogenic properties of ephedrine/methylxanthine mixtures: Human studies. *Int. J. Obes.* 10:467–81, 1986.
10. Astrup, A., et al. The effect of ephedrine/caffeine mixture on energy expenditure and body composition in obese women. *Metabolism* 41:686–88, 1992.

11. Mctavish, D., and Heel, R. C. Dexfenfluramine. A review of its pharmacological properties and therapeutic potential in obesity. *Drugs* 43:713–33, 1992.

12. Breuhm, L. Comparison of an ephedrine/caffeine combination and dexfenfluramine in the treatment of obesity. A double-blind multi-centered trial in general practice. *Int. I. Obes.* 18:99–103, 1994.

13. American Pharmaceutical Association. *Handbook of Nonprescription Drugs,* 8th ed. American Pharmaceutical Association, Washington, D.C., 1986.

14. Tinkelman, D. G., and Avner, S. E. Ephedrine therapy in asthmatic children. *JAMA* 237:553–57, 1977.

15. Daly, P. A., et al. Ephedrine, caffeine and aspirin: safety and efficacy for treatment of human obesity. *Int. J. Obes.* 17 (suppl. 1): S73–78, 1993.

16. Weil, J., et al. Prophylactic aspirin and risk of peptic ulcer bleeding. *BMJ* 310:827–30, 1995.

Chapter 7: Other Natural Weight Loss Promoters

1. Spiller, G. A. *Dietary fiber in health and nutrition.* CRC Press, Boca Raton, Fla., 1994.

2. Bjorntorp, P., and Brodoff, B. N. *Obesity.* J. B. Lippincott Company, Philadelphia, 1992.

3. Halama, W. H., and Maudlin, J. L. Distal esophageal obstruction due to a guar gum preparation. *South. Med. J.* 85:642–46, 1992.

4. Henry, C. A., et al. Glucomannan and risk of oesophageal obstruction. *BMJ* 292:591–92, 1986.

5. Krotkiewski, M. Effect of guar on body weight, hunger ratings and metabolism in obese subjects. *Clinical Science* 66:329–6, 1984.

6. Krotkiewski, M., and Smith, U. Dietary fibre in obesity. In *Dietary Fiber Perspectives. Reviews and Bibliography*, ed. Leeds, A. R., and Avenell, A. John Libbey, London, 1985, pp. 61–7.

7. Krotkiewski, M. Effect of guar gum on body-weight, hunger ratings

and metabolism in obese subjects. *Br. J. Nutr.* 52:97–105, 1984.

8. Anonymous. Better than oat bran. *Science News* 145:28, 1994.

9. Walsh, D. E., Yaghoubian, V., and Behforooz, A. Effect of glucomannan on obese patients: A clinical study. *Int. J. Obes.* 8:289–93, 1984.

10. Biancardi, G., Palmiero, L., and Ghirardi, P. E. Glucomannan in the treatment of overweight patients with osteoarthrosis. *Curr. Ther. Res.* 46:908–12, 1989.

11. El-Shebini, S. M., et al. The role of pectin as a slimming agent. *J. Clin. Biochem. Nutr.* 4:255–62, 1988.

12. Solum, T. T., et al. The influence of a high-fibre diet on body weight, serum lipids and blood pressure in slightly overweight persons. A randomized, double-blind, placebo-controlled investigation with diet and fibre tablets (DumoVital). *Int. J. Obes.* 11 (Suppl. 1): 67–71, 1987.

13. Ryttig, K. R., Larsen, S., and Haegh, L. Treatment of slightly to moderately overweight persons: A double-blind placebo-controlled investigation with diet and fibre tablets (DumoVital). *Tidsskr Nor Laegeforen* 104:989–91, 1984.

14. Rossner, S., et al. Weight reduction with dietary fibre supplements. Results of two double-blind studies. *Acta Med. Scand.* 222:83–8, 1987.

15. Ryttig, K. R., et al. A dietary fibre supplement and weight maintenance after weight reduction: A randomized, double-blind, placebo-controlled long-term trial. *Int. J. Obes.* 14:763–9, 1989.

16. Rigaud, D., et al. Mild overweight treated with energy restriction and a dietary fiber supplement: A 6-month randomized, double-blind, placebo-controlled trial. *Int. J. Obes.* 14:763–9, 1990.

17. Nomura, F., et al. Liver function in moderate obesity—study in 534 moderately obese subjects among 4613 male company employees. *Int. J. Obes.* 10:349–54, 1986.

18. Dean, D. H., and Hiramoto, R. N. Weight loss during pancreatin feeding of rats. *Nutrition Reports International* 29:167–72, 1984.

19. Baba, N., Bracco, E. F., and Hashim, S. A. Enhanced thermogenesis

and diminished deposition of fat in response to overfeeding with diet containing medium chain triglyceride. *Am. J. Clin. Nutr.* 35: 678–82, 1982.

20. Hill, J. O., et al. Thermogenesis in humans during overfeeding with medium-chain triglycerides in man. *Amer. J. Clin. Nutr.* 44:630–34, 1986.

21. Hill, J. O., et al. Thermogenesis in man during overfeeding with medium chain triglycerides. *Metabolism* 38:641–48, 1989.

22. Seaton, T. B., et al. Thermic effect of medium-chain and long-chain triglycerides in man. *Am. J. Clin. Nutr.* 44:630–84, 1986.

23. Chee, H., Romsos, D. R., and Leveille, G. A. Influence of (−)−hydroxycitrate on lipogenesis in chickens and rats. *J. Nutr.* 107:112–19, 1977.

    Sullivan, A. C., et al. Effect of (−)−hydroxycitrate upon the accumulation of lipid in the rat. I. Lipogenesis. *Lipids* 9:121–28, 1974.

24. Rao, R. N., and Sakariah, K. K. Lipid-lowering and antiobesity effect of (−)−hydroxycitric acid. *Nutr. Res.* 8:209–12, 1988.

25. van Gaal, L., et al. Exploratory study of coenzyme Q10 in obesity. In *Biomedical and Clinical Aspects of Coenzyme Q*, ed. Folkers, K., and Yamamura, Y. vol. 4 Elsevier Science Publ., Amsterdam, 1984, pp. 369–73.

26. Drenick, E. J. Exogenous thyroid hormones to accelerate weight loss. *Obesity Bariatric Med.* 4:244–50, 1975.

    Abraham, G. K., et al. The effects of triiodothyronine on energy expenditure, nitrogen balance and rates of weight and fat loss in obese patients during prolonged caloric restriction. *Int. J. Obes.* 9: 433–42, 1985.

    Rozen, R., et al. Effects of a "physiological" dose of triiodothyronine on obese subjects during a protein-sparing diet. *Int. J. Obes.* 10:303–12, 1986.

Index

Index

blood pressure, 107
    exercise and, 84, 92
    high, 3, 9, 16–17, 92, 114, 115
    lowering of, 10, 116
brain, 23, 107, 112
    fat cells and, 6, 8
breads, Healthy Exchange list for, 49–53
breakfast, 70–71
brown fat, 11–13
butter, 60

caffeine, ephedrine with, 106, 108–113, 115–116
calories, 33–42
    in cereals, 71
    excess, in lean vs. overweight individuals, 12–13
    in fruits, 74–75
    Healthy Exchange recommendations for different intakes of, 37–42
    in legumes, 71–72
    muscle vs. fat and, 85
    in vegetables, 75, 79
    wasting of, *see* diet-induced thermogenesis
    weight and, 5, 6, 12–13
cancer, 14, 16, 43, 45, 47, 50, 59, 60
carbohydrates:
    complex, 28–30, 32, 49–53
    in diet, 28–30, 43, 49–53
    metabolism of, 7, 29
    percentage of, 32
    refined, 7, 32
carbon dioxide, 84
carnitine, 130–131
casein, 66, 135
cataracts, 47
cell membranes, 59, 61–62
cereals:
    breakfast, 70–71
    calories and fiber in, 71
    Healthy Exchange list for, 49–53

cheese, Healthy Exchange list for, 67–69
chervil, fresh, baked potato salad with, 51–52
chick-pea salad with red onion and mustard greens, 72–73
children:
    diabetes in, 17
    obesity in, viii, 84
China, pickled vegetables in, 45
cholesterol, 10, 59, 116, 130
    exercise and, 84
    HDL, 60, 102
    high, 9, 17, 59
    LDL, 60, 64
chromium, 98–105, 138
coenzyme Q10, 130–131
colon cancer, 50
corticosteroids (cortisol), 99

depression, 5, 86, 87, 114
D-fenfluramine, 112–113
diabetes, 3, 7, 14, 16, 99, 114, 115
    chromium and, 102
    diet and, 28–30, 50, 59
    type I (insulin-dependent), 17
    type II (non-insulin-dependent), 9–10, 17–19, 61–62
diet, dieting:
    American, 14
    food intake restricted by, ix, 1, 5, 27
    guidelines for, 27–82
    high-complex-carbohydrate, high-fiber (HCF), 28–30
    high-fat, viii, 9, 13–14, 29–30
    high-fiber, low-calorie, 27–28
    Japanese, 13–14
    liquid protein, ix
    low-fat, 29, 30
    poor, 9, 10
    of pregnant women, 2
    weight-loss tips and, 28
    yo-yo effect and, 1, 7, 8

Index

Index

Index

Index